T0358579

Sharon A. Gutman, PhD, OTR

Brain Injury and Gender Role Strain: Rebuilding Adult Lifestyles After Injury

Brain Injury and Gender Role Strain: Rebuilding Adult Lifestyles After Injury has been co-published simultaneously as *Occupational Therapy in Mental Health,* Volume 15, Numbers 3/4 2000.

Pre-publication REVIEWS, COMMENTARIES, EVALUATIONS . . .

"**S**haron Gutman helps to bring a new richness to the professional literature in occupational therapy with her deft study of the implications for practice of an important cultural factor: gender identity. Her depiction of the pre- and post-morbid experiences of four men in an adult intervention program for people with brain injury is sensitively drawn. She shows most effectively why it is important for occupational therapists to maintain a holistic approach to everyday activities in naturally-occurring contexts. Readers of this book will be familiar with the independent living and disability rights philosophy that defines disability as the result more of social, physical, and legal barriers to performance than of a biomedical impairment itself. Gutman's attention to the impact of dysfunction on the performance of everyday occupations more than amply shows how lifting the barriers to a more engaged lifestyle (including man-sized helpings of male-identified social activities, caring male mentorship, and work experiences) can make for a more rewarding existence and the resumption of a trajectory of adult development among men with brain injury. Gutman's sensitivity to the individual differences among these four men, as well as the commonalities of their experience as a result of their disability, opens new avenues of perception."

Gelya Frank, PhD

Author of *Venus on Wheels: Two Decades of Dialogue on Disability, Biography, and Being Female in America*

"*L*ittle attention has been devoted to the development of intervention strategies for use with individuals with traumatic brain injury (TBI) in the postacute period of recovery. Dr. Gutman has developed an innovative target setting and treatment planning protocol that focuses the therapist on the key areas of concern for individuals in the postacute period of recovery from TBI.

Many individuals are injured during the transition from adolescent roles to mature adult roles. Goals, activities, and rites of passage are therefore missed by these individuals. Long cherished goals suddenly appear unavailable. Activities that might appear important to therapists are stripped of their meaning for the client leading to lack of motivation and resistance.

Through extensive quotations the reader gets to understand the circumstances and concerns of each client. Dr. Gutman's work encourages therapists to set their rehabilitative interventions in the context of the development of meaningful life structures for persons with TBI. The detailed presentation of four individuals demonstrates how the concept of chronic role strain assisted the therapist to form goals and treatment interventions. Through this

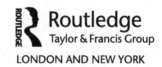

LONDON AND NEW YORK

Brain Injury and Gender Role Strain: Rebuilding Adult Lifestyles After Injury

Brain Injury and Gender Role Strain: Rebuilding Adult Lifestyles After Injury has been co-published simultaneously as *Occupational Therapy in Mental Health*, Volume 15, Numbers 3/4 2000.

The *Occupational Therapy in Mental Health* Monographic "Separates"

Below is a list of "separates," which in serials librarianship means a special issue simultaneously published as a special journal issue or double-issue *and* as a "separate" hardbound monograph. (This is a format which we also call a "DocuSerial.")

"Separates" are published because specialized libraries or professionals may wish to purchase a specific thematic issue by itself in a format which can be separately cataloged and shelved, as opposed to purchasing the journal on an on-going basis. Faculty members may also more easily consider a "separate" for classroom adoption.

"Separates" are carefully classified separately with the major book jobbers so that the journal tie-in can be noted on new book order slips to avoid duplicate purchasing.

You may wish to visit Haworth's website at . . .

http://www.haworthpressinc.com

. . . to search our online catalog for complete tables of contents of these separates and related publications.

You may also call 1-800-HAWORTH (outside US/Canada: 607-722-5857), or Fax 1-800-895-0582 (outside US/Canada: 607-771-0012), or e-mail at:

getinfo@haworthpressinc.com

Brain Injury and Gender Role Strain: Rebuilding Adult Lifestyles After Injury, by Sharon A. Gutman, PhD, OTR (Vol. 15, No. 3/4, 2000). *"Dr. Gutman has developed an innovative target setting and treatment planning protocol that focuses the therapist on the key areas of concern. I highly recommend this book to therapists who work with clients in the post-acute period of recovery from TBI." (Gordon Muir Giles, MA, Dip COT, OTR, Director of Neurobehavioral Services, Crestwood Behavioral Health, Inc., and Assistant Professor, Samuel Merritt College, Oakland, California)*

New Frontiers in Psychosocial Occupational Therapy, edited by Anne Hiller Scott, PhD, OTR, FAOTA (Vol. 14, No. 1/2, 1998). *"Speaks a clear message about mental health practice in occupational therapy, shattering old visions of practice to insights about empowerment and advocacy." (Sharan L. Schwartzberg, EdD, OTR, FAOTA, Professor and Chair, Boston School of Occupational Therapy, Tufts University)*

Evaluation and Treatment of the Psychogeriatric Patient, edited by Diane Gibson, MS, OTR (Vol. 10, No. 3, 1991). *"Occupational therapists everywhere, learners and sophisticates alike, and in-hospital and out-patient areas as well as home-bound and home-active, would enjoy and profit from this exposition as much as I did." (American Association of Psychiatric Administrators)*

Student Recruitment in Psychosocial Occupational Therapy: Intergenerational Approaches, edited by Susan Haiman (Vol. 10, No. 1, 1990). *"Can serve to enlighten both academics and clinicians as to their roles in attracting students to become practitioners in mental health settings. Each article could well serve as a catalyst for discussion in the classroom or clinic." (Canadian Journal of Occupational Therapy)*

Group Protocols: A Psychosocial Compendium, edited by Susan Haiman (Vol. 9, No. 4, 1990). *"Presents succinct protocols for a wide range of groups that are typically run by activities therapists, vocational counselors, art therapists, and other mental health professionals." (International Journal of Group Psychotherapy)*

Instrument Development in Occupational Therapy, edited by Janet Hawkins Watts and Chestina Brollier (Vol. 8, No. 4, 1989). *Examines content and concurrent validity and development of the Assessment of Occupational Functioning (AOF), and carefully compares the AOF with a similar instrument, the Occupational Case Analysis Interview and Rating Scale (OCAIRS), to discover the similarities and strengths of these instruments.*

Group Process and Structure in Psychosocial Occupational Therapy, edited by Diane Gibson, MS, OTR (Vol. 8, No. 3, 1989). *Highly skilled professionals examine the important concepts of group therapy to help build cohesive, safe groups.*

Treatment of Substance Abuse: Psychosocial Occupational Therapy Approaches, edited by Diane Gibson, MS, OTR (Vol. 8, No. 2, 1989). *A unique overview of contemporary assessment and rehabilitation of alcohol and chemical dependent substance abusers.*

The Development of Standardized Clinical Evaluations in Mental Health, Principal Investigator: Noomi Katz, PhD, OTR; edited by Claudia Kay Allen, MA, OTR, FAOTA; Commentator: Janice P. Burke, MA, OTR, FAOTA (Vol. 8, No. 1, 1988). *"Contains a collection of research-based articles encompassing several evaluations that can be used by occupational therapists practicing in mental health."* (*American Journal of Occupational Therapy*)

Evaluation and Treatment of Adolescents and Children, edited by Diane Gibson, MS, OTR (Vol. 7, No. 2, 1987). *Experts share research results and practices that have proven successful in helping young people who suffer from psychiatric and medical disorders.*

Treatment of the Chronic Schizophrenic Patient, edited by Diane Gibson, MS, OTR (Vol. 6, No. 2, 1986). *"Reflect[s] creative and fresh concepts of current treatment for the chronically mentally ill. . . . Recommended for the therapist practicing in psychiatry."* (*Canadian Journal of Occupational Therapy*)

The Evaluation and Treatment of Eating Disorders, edited by Diane Gibson, MS, OTR (Vol. 6, No. 1, 1986). *"A wealth of information. . . . Covers the subject thoroughly. . . . This book, well-conceived and well-written, is recommended not only for clinicians working with clients with anorexia nervosa and bulimia but for all therapists who wish to become acquainted with the subject of eating disorders in general."* (*Library Journal*)

Philosophical and Historical Roots of Occupational Therapy, edited by Karen Diasio Serrett (Vol. 5, No. 3, 1985). *"Recommended as an easy-to-get-through background read for occupational therapists and for generalists wishing a fuller acquaintance with the backdrop of occupational therapy."* (*Rehabilitation Literature*)

Short-Term Treatment in Occupational Therapy, edited by Diane Gibson, MS, OTR, and Kathy Kaplan, MS, OTR (Vol. 4, No. 3, 1984). *"Thought provoking and relevant to various issues facing OTs in a short term inpatient psychiatric setting. . . . Very readable . . . concise, well-written, and stimulating."* (*Canadian Journal of Occupational Therapy*)

SCORE: Solving Community Obstacles and Restoring Employment, by Lynn Wechsler Kramer, MS, OTR (Vol. 4, No. 1, 1984). *"This needed book is an effective instrument for occupational therapists wanting to 'teach employable handicapped how to obtain a job in a competitive (labor) market.' Very relevant to professional practice . . . a useful how-to instrument."* (*The American Journal of Occupational Therapy*)

Occupational Therapy with Borderline Patients, edited by Diane Gibson, MS, OTR (Vol. 3, No. 3, 1983). *"Offers clinicians an opportunity to review current theoretical concepts, management, and design of activity groups for this population. Well written . . . provides good reference lists and well-developed discussions."* (*The American Journal of Occupational Therapy*)

Psychiatric Occupational Therapy in the Army, edited by LTC Paul D. Ellsworth, MPH, OTR, FAOTA, and Diane Gibson, MS, OTR (Vol. 3, No. 2, 1983). *This unique volume focuses on the historical contributions, current trends, and future directions of army occupational therapists practicing in the military mental health arena.*

Brain Injury and Gender Role Strain: Rebuilding Adult Lifestyles After Injury

Sharon A. Gutman, PhD, OTR

Brain Injury and Gender Role Strain: Rebuilding Adult Lifestyles After Injury has been co-published simultaneously as *Occupational Therapy in Mental Health*, Volume 15, Numbers 3/4 2000.

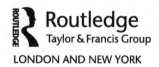

Routledge
Taylor & Francis Group

LONDON AND NEW YORK

Brain Injury and Gender Role Strain: Rebuilding Adult Lifestyles After Injury has been co-published simultaneously as *Occupational Therapy in Mental Health*™, Volume 15, Numbers 3/4 2000.

First published 2000 by The Haworth Press, Inc.

2 Park Square, Milton Park, Abingdon, Oxfordshire OX14 4RN
605 Third Avenue, New York, NY 10017

Routledge is an imprint of the Taylor & Francis Group, an informa business

First issued in hardback 2020

Cover design by Thomas J. Mayshock Jr.

Library of Congress Cataloging-in-Publication Data

Gutman, Sharon A.
    Brain injury and gender role strain : rebuilding adult lifestyles after injury / Sharon A. Gutman.
       p. cm.
    "Co-published simultaneously as Occupational therapy in mental health, volume 15, numbers 3/4 2000."
    Includes bibliographical references and index.
    1. Brain damage–Patients–Rehabilitation. 2. Occupational therapy. 3. Gender role. I. Occupational therapy in mental health. II. Title.
RC387.5 .G88 2000
616.8′03–dc21   00-058210

ISBN 13: 978-0-7890-1186-2 (hbk)
ISBN 13: 978-0-789-01187-9 (pbk)

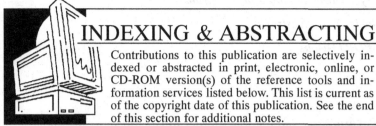

INDEXING & ABSTRACTING

Contributions to this publication are selectively indexed or abstracted in print, electronic, online, or CD-ROM version(s) of the reference tools and information services listed below. This list is current as of the copyright date of this publication. See the end of this section for additional notes.

- *Abstracts in Social Gerontology: Current Literature on Aging*

- *Alzheimer's Disease Education & Referral Center (ADEAR)*

- *BUBL Information Service: An Internet-based Information Service for the UK higher education community <URL: http://bubl.ac.uk/>*

- *CINAHL (Cumulative Index to Nursing & Allied Health Literature), in print, also on CD-ROM from CD PLUS, EBSCO, and SilverPlatter, and online from CDP Online (formerly BRS), Data-Star, and PaperChase. (Support materials include Subject Heading List, Database Search Guide, and instructional video.)*

- *CNPIEC Reference Guide: Chinese National Directory of Foreign Periodicals*

- *Developmental Medicine & Child Neurology*

- *EMBASE/Excerpta Medica Secondary Publishing Division <URL: http://elsevier.nl>*

- *Exceptional Child Education Resources (ECER) (CD/ROM from SilverPlatter and hard copy)*

- *Family Studies Database (online and CD/ROM)*

- *FINDEX <www.publist.com>*

- *Mental Health Abstracts (online through DIALOG)*

- *Occupational Therapy Database (OTDBASE) <www.otdbase.com>*

- *Occupational Therapy Index*

- *OT BibSys*

- *PASCAL, c/o Institute de L'Information Scientifique et Technique <http://www.inist.fr>*

(continued)

- *Psychiatric Rehabilitation Journal*
- *Social Work Abstracts*
- *SPORTDiscus*

Special Bibliographic Notes related to special journal issues (separates) and indexing/abstracting:

- indexing/abstracting services in this list will also cover material in any "separate" that is co-published simultaneously with Haworth's special thematic journal issue or DocuSerial. Indexing/abstracting usually covers material at the article/chapter level.
- monographic co-editions are intended for either non-subscribers or libraries which intend to purchase a second copy for their circulating collections.
- monographic co-editions are reported to all jobbers/wholesalers/approval plans. The source journal is listed as the "series" to assist the prevention of duplicate purchasing in the same manner utilized for books-in-series.
- to facilitate user/access services all indexing/abstracting services are encouraged to utilize the co-indexing entry note indicated at the bottom of the first page of each article/chapter/contribution.
- this is intended to assist a library user of any reference tool (whether print, electronic, online, or CD-ROM) to locate the monographic version if the library has purchased this version but not a subscription to the source journal.
- individual articles/chapters in any Haworth publication are also available through the Haworth Document Delivery Service (HDDS).

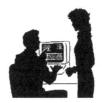

I dedicate this book to my parents, Evelyn and Jesse.

ABOUT THE AUTHOR

Sharon A. Gutman, PhD, OTR, is Assistant Professor at Long Island University where she teaches and conducts research in the Division of Occupational Therapy. She earned her PhD in Occupational Therapy and Rehabilitation Research at New York University. She has practiced occupational therapy for approximately 10 years and has specialized in traumatic brain injury rehabilitation for eight years. Dr. Gutman has practiced in both sub-acute and long-term brain injury rehabilitation for people with moderate to severe brain injury who are reintegrating into community settings, returning to work, and rebuilding social relationships. Dr. Gutman has published a number of research articles regarding long-term brain injury sequelae and the effectiveness of brain injury intervention methods.

Brain Injury and Gender Role Strain: Rebuilding Adult Lifestyles After Injury

CONTENTS

Acknowledgments

I thank Mary V. Donohue, PhD, OT, FAOTA, Jim Hinojosa, PhD, OT, FAOTA, Dawn Leger, PhD, Marie Louise Blount, AM, OT, FAOTA, Anne Hiller Scott, PhD, OTR, FAOTA, Winnifred Olivaria, Chris Rosner, PhD, RN, Ellen Greer, MA, OTR, Pat Gentile, MS, OTR, and Marianne Mortera, MS, OTR. I also thank the men who participated in the intervention and who generously shared their lives with me for one summer. This book was derived from research completed for my doctoral degree at New York University. I thank the American Occupational Therapy Foundation for a grant that made this research possible.

Chapter 1

Introduction:
"I Never Thought This Is How My Life
Would Turn Out"

John was a high school senior who was planning to attend an out-of-state college in the following fall. It was late May and he was finishing school projects and preparing to take final examinations. A number of students were caught up in the frenzy of graduation and graduation parties. It seemed that every weekend a graduation party was annoying neighbors, worrying parents, and causing increased concern for the local police department. Statistically, this is the time of year when most auto vehicle accidents occur in the 16-21 year old age group (Brain Injury Association, 1997; Francell & Snell, 1999).

John was a well-liked gregarious student who excelled in hockey, soccer, and wrestling. He was an average B student who was thought to be highly intelligent by his teachers, but lacked discipline and study habits. Instead, John devoted much of his time to sports and partying–particularly as this was his last year of high school and he had already been accepted into a private liberal arts college in the northeastern United States. This college had a Health Science School where John planned to become a physical therapist and specialize in sports injuries.

On the night of May 16 John left his parent's home at 8:00 p.m. to attend a graduation party at the home of a young girl, Patti, whom he

---

[Haworth co-indexing entry note]: "Introduction: 'I Never Thought This Is How My Life Would Turn Out.'" Gutman, Sharon A. Co-published simultaneously in *Occupational Therapy in Mental Health* (The Haworth Press, Inc.) Vol. 15, No. 3/4, 2000, pp. 1-11; and: *Brain Injury and Gender Role Strain: Rebuilding Adult Lifestyles After Injury* (Sharon A. Gutman) The Haworth Press, Inc., 2000, pp. 1-11. Single or multiple copies of this article are available for a fee from The Haworth Document Delivery Service [1-800-342-9678, 9:00 a.m. - 5:00 p.m. (EST). E-mail address: getinfo@haworthpressinc.com].

grew up with since childhood. John's parents felt reassured that he was going to Patti's house, as the two sets of parents were old trusted friends from college. But Patti's parents had made a last minute, emergency flight to Florida to attend to Patti's grandmother who had just sustained a stroke.

When John arrived at Patti's party, the house had already become crowded and smoke-filled with cigarettes, marijuana, and the smell of alcohol. The sounds of loud music drifted from the house into the warm air of summer and through the neighborhood streets. John could hear his friends splashing in the backyard pool as he went into the living room and reached for a small bottle of beer lying amongst several large kegs. John says that he can't remember anything else about that night. But John's friends' stories in the police report fill in the missing pieces of information.

After arriving at the party John began to drink heavily with four of his soccer buddies. They began to become abusive, vomiting on Patti's parents' carpet, physically pushing and threatening some of the other males at the party, and grabbing Patti when she tried to stop them. John and three of his soccer buddies took Patti and they left her parents' house. John was driving with Patti in the front passenger seat. The three guys in the backseat were so loud that John could not hear the other cars on the street. Patti could see that John was having trouble understanding the traffic signals and pleaded with him to slow down and let her drive. John didn't see that the traffic light was red. The police report determined that the car was speeding at 58 mph in a 25 mile residential zone. John swerved to miss an oncoming car and crashed into a telephone pole. Two of the males in the backseat died, the third survived with a broken leg and arm, and a minor contusion. Patti was the only one of the five who had worn her seatbelt but still sustained a broken collarbone and severe nerve impingement throughout her neck and right brachial plexus. John's head hit the windshield causing his brain to bounce back and forth within his skull, thus shearing and bruising cortical tissue. He sustained dorsolateral frontal lobe impairment, left parietal damage, and a cerebellar lesion. The five were rushed to a local community hospital that was not equipped to handle the acute crisis of traumatic brain injury. John was placed on a ventilator to breathe. His blood pressure had dropped precariously low causing the circulation of oxygenated blood to his brain to slow down.

All the while, cerebrospinal fluid was increasing in his brain, impinging upon cortical tissue.

After 24 hours John's parents transferred him to an urban city hospital that specialized in the acute care of traumatic brain injury. Here John underwent a ventriculostomy in which a small tube was inserted into his brain to relieve the increasing cerebrospinal fluid. John was also given medications to raise his blood pressure so that oxygenated blood would flow to his brain. After five days John continued to remain in a comatose state despite the fact that his intracranial pressure had dropped to a normal level. His parents grew increasingly frightened as they began to recognize the severity of John's condition. They questioned the doctors who could not give them specific answers, only stating that, at this time, it was impossible to know how much John would recover. Instead, the doctors spoke in technical terms that were difficult for John's parents to comprehend, "John had sustained cerebral contusions to his left frontal and parietal regions, and cerebellar damage as a result of the car accident. John was in a comatose state in which his brain stem had been spared but at the cost of severe cortical damage." This, John's parents were informed, "offered a better prognosis than if John's brain stem was damaged, thus leaving him in a persistent vegetative state." But to John's parents, they couldn't imagine a worse condition than the one John presently appeared to be in.

At ten days John began to open his eyes and respond to painful stimuli (for example, being pinched) but did not respond to his name or to people in his immediate environment. This was a very difficult period of time for his parents, as John appeared to be conscious–his eyes were opened–but he was unable to recognize or interact with anyone. Moreover he was fed through a nasogastric tube that was inserted into his stomach and he urinated through a catheter into a clear plastic bag tied to his hospital bed. To John's mother he appeared like a body without a soul and she prayed every night for God to return her son to her.

At 14 days John began to track objects with his eyes and could blink to indicate yes or no. He could recognize his family members and began to recognize the faces of his therapists, nurses, and physicians. At 16 days John began to identify objects and familiar faces with one-word verbalizations. While the right side of his body was largely immobile as a result of muscle spasticity (i.e., abnormally increased muscle tone), John was beginning to use his left arm to reach for different colored balls and self-care items that the occupational therapist would ask him to grasp. He began to spend greater periods of time sitting upright in his hospital bed or in the chair in his room. The therapist told John that he would begin to learn wheelchair ambulation during the next week.

John would spend 5 months in the hospital relearning basic skills such as talking, eating, walking, toileting, bathing, and dressing. The speech therapist helped John to learn how to vocalize words and put sentences together in a correct sequence. The occupational therapist and speech therapist together helped John to learn to eat again without aspirating (choking). Both therapists also helped John to use a memory and schedule book to enhance his memory by recording the day's events, physician appointments, and field trips outside of the hospital where John began to relearn community skills–for example, shopping for groceries, banking, negotiating traffic signals in a wheelchair. The occupational therapist also helped John to prepare for eventual community living by relearning independent living skills such as money management, bill paying, and preparing meals. John and his occupational therapist also made his home environment safer by installing grab bars, wheelchair ramps, non-scald showerheads, and lights that turn on when movement is sensed. The occupational therapist also reprogrammed John's personal computer to cue John to wake-up, go through his morning self-care routine, and prepare breakfast. John's physical therapist helped him to regain joint movement, muscular strength, and physical endurance. His vocational counselor helped John to regain basic work skills and study habits for a possible return to school.

At the end of John's five-month hospital rehabilitation period he returned home to live with his parents. Without the structured schedule of the rehabilitation hospital and the motivation of his therapists, John became increasingly depressed and isolated. He had not fully understood the severity of his physical and cognitive injuries when he was discharged from the hospital and assumed that he would attend college in the fall with his friends. John's severe short-term memory loss, poor concentration, and decreased frustration tolerance made it unlikely that he could successfully live away from home and attend the competitive out-of-state college he had been accepted to last fall. After seven months of living at home–one year after his accident–John was severely depressed, often slept throughout the day, rarely bathed, and began drinking heavily with several former high school acquaintances who brought him alcohol.

John's parents decided that they could no longer handle his problems alone and sought assistance. They hoped that John could benefit from a community-based residential program for young adults who sustained traumatic brain injury (TBI). John was placed in a 24 hour supervised community group home with four other males between the ages of 18-40, and one female who was 20 years old. John was resistant to living at this facility and frequently stated that he felt "even more like a misfit being here." In his first month at the residential TBI facility he told his case manager that his life ended the night of his accident.

> I wish I had died with the other guys. People say I'm the lucky one cause I made it through. But look at this life. Maybe it's my punishment for killing them [the two boys who died in the car accident]. I got no one. No girlfriend; what girl would want me? I got no friends. I got no purpose in life. No job, no education. This isn't the life I pictured when I thought about me in the future. Now what future do I have to look forward to?

John's experience of traumatic brain injury is fairly typical. Eighty percent of individuals who sustain TBI are young males between the ages of 18-30. They largely sustain head injury through risk-taking activities: driving while intoxicated, engaging in violence–often under the influence of alcohol–and participating in sports having a safety risk element. Young men like John, who sustain TBI between the years of 18-30, find that head injury severely disrupts the transition from adolescence to adulthood. These young men are often left alone to make the transition from adolescent to adult roles in a society that rigidly defines masculinity through specific male gender roles. Social roles such as husband/boyfriend, father, son, worker, sports participant, and friend are male gender roles that are often difficult to form and maintain post-TBI due to the physical, cognitive, and psychosocial sequlae of TBI (Brain Injury Association, 1997; Gutman, 1997, 1999; Merritt, 1999; Schmidt, Garvin, Heinemann, & Kelly, 1995). When the gender roles and activities–once used to support their pre-injury gender identity–are no longer available, *gender role strain* often occurs.

GENDER ROLE STRAIN

Gender role strain is a feeling reported by men with disabilities, such as TBI, that they are unable to attain the lifestyle and roles of an adult man in their society. Gender role strain describes the experience of men who perceive their internal personality traits to be congruent with their personal expectations of masculinity, but who–as a result of traumatic disability–feel denied access to male roles in the larger society. Males with TBI who used pre-injury masculine gender social roles and activities to express their masculine gender identity, commonly report post-injury gender role strain if they are unable to presently engage in those roles and activities. Such males express frustration regarding unsuccessful personal attempts to achieve self-perceived masculine adult roles–for example, worker/economic provider, spouse/sexual partner, and parent. Often, as length of time post-injury increases, participation in masculine gender social roles and activities decreases. Males with TBI frequently become socially isolated after injury, refrain from participation in pre-injury masculine gender social roles and activities, and fail to rebuild pre-injury relationships that support their male gender identity (Brown & Vandergoot, 1998; Gutman & Napier-Klemic, 1996).

Gender role strain can be particularly problematic for young men who sustain their TBI between the ages of 18-30, as these are the years in human development when the expression of one's gender role through adult worker roles and dating/courtship activities becomes a primary maturational task (Erikson, 1950; Levinson, 1978; Merritt, 1999). Males who sustain TBI in this period of time may feel ill-equipped to adopt the roles and activities of adult males as a result of sequelae (i.e., residual deficits) secondary to injury. The sustained stress resulting from unsuccessful attempts to transition from adolescent to adult male roles–exacerbated by inadequate coping strategies–are believed to be primary factors contributing to depression, anxiety, decreased motivation, and low self-esteem in men with TBI. Men with TBI who experience gender role strain report feeling unable to achieve the status of an adult male in western society (Gutman, 1997, 1999; Rosenthal, Christensen, & Ross, 1998).

Researchers suggest that adult males with TBI experience disruption in gender role enactment as more problematic than females (Gutman & Napier-Klemic, 1996; Moore, Stambrook, & Gill, 1994;

Schmidt et al., 1995). Females tend to independently seek greater social support after TBI than do males. Such social support often translates into decreased isolation, greater attainment of emotional and material resources and enhanced community reintegration. Females also more commonly re-establish post-injury participation in most of their pre-injury gender social roles and activities than do males. Conversely, male participation in pre-injury gender social roles and activities tends to decrease as length of time post-injury increases.

Several reasons may account for this difference found between males and females regarding the ability to re-establish gender roles after TBI. One reason may relate to the way in which females in western society are culturally socialized to establish social connections that provide emotional and material support. In times of crisis–such as the onset of chronic disability–the opportunity to rely on others to provide support may be critical in the successful adjustment to disability. Males who are traditionally socialized to refrain from help-seeking behaviors and who tend to isolate themselves in crisis, may be less likely to avail themselves of pre-injury social support and fail to re-establish participation in pre-injury gender social roles and activities (Jordan, Kaplan, Miller, Stiver, & Surrey, 1991; Kaschak, 1992).

A second reason accounting for this male/female distinction in post-TBI gender role enactment may relate to differences in the ways that males and females use social roles and activities to express gender identity. While females characteristically express gender identity through intimate social relationships based on a sense of caring and connection, males traditionally express gender identity through roles that serve economic or physical functions, such as worker, spouse, economic provider to offspring, and sports participant (Jordan et al., 1991). Such male gender social roles are often lost and difficult to re-establish after TBI due to physical, cognitive, and psychosocial sequelae (Gomez-Hernandez, Max, Kosier, Paradiso, & Robinson, 1997; Trombly, Radomski, & Davis, 1998).

Additionally, because western males may be culturally socialized to refrain from help-seeking in crisis, they may be more susceptible than females to social isolation and gender role strain post-TBI. Males may also believe that participation in traditionally masculine gender roles alone can provide a sense of gender role satisfaction, and thus fail to engage in post-injury gender-neutral social roles and activities that may provide adequate masculine role expression.

However, while researchers have identified the existence of male gender role strain after TBI, little effort has been put forth to apply such knowledge to clinical intervention methods. In fact much of the treatment addressing TBI has been concentrated on acute and sub-acute care–in other words, the first eight months of recovery when physical injuries take precedence over psychosocial issues. Ironically, researchers have found through long-term follow-up studies, that clients and their families experience the psychosocial stress of TBI as more debilitating than the clients' physical impairments (Brzuzy & Speziale, 1997; Burleigh, Farber, & Gillard, 1998; Mazaux et al., 1997).

Health care professionals have begun to more frequently identify and treat the long-term psychosocial sequelae of TBI. Psychologists often assist individuals with TBI to alleviate depression and enhance behavioral skill. Vocational counselors help individuals to regain work skills and to obtain employment or volunteer work. Occupational therapists assist clients to relearn activities of daily living–such as dressing, bathing, and meal preparation–and community skills: use of public transportation, community shopping, and money management. While these skills are important functional abilities, they are also abilities that health care professionals and family members–rather than clients–identify as most meaningful. Studies in which clients identified their most troubling post-injury problems revealed that males 2+ years post-TBI report feeling unable to engage in the common culture-specific, gender social roles and activities characteristic of their particular adult life stage. The inability to participate in the social roles and activities of male adulthood is a primary characteristic of gender role strain. Decreased opportunities to socialize, loss of significant relationships–such as, spousal and parental roles–isolation and loneliness, inability to regain employment, and a decline in occupational status are long-term sequelae commonly reported by males having sustained TBI. Adult males with TBI may feel unable to re-enter their adult culture in ways they find personally meaningful (Burleigh et al., 1998; Bowen, Neumann, Conner, Tennant, & Chamberlain, 1998; Corrigan, Smith-Knapp, & Granger, 1998).

Commonly available rehabilitation services for males with TBI–behavioral management, cognitive retraining, and community skill training–may not effectively alleviate gender role strain. In an effort to provide more appropriate therapy services for males experiencing post-TBI gender role strain, I developed a set of guidelines for practice based on my clinical experience and review of pertinent research and theory. The set of guidelines is designed to alleviate gender role strain by helping men with TBI to rebuild desired roles and activities of male adulthood in accordance with their own perceptions of adult male lifestyles.

MY EXPERIENCE AS A THERAPIST IN TRAUMATIC BRAIN INJURY REHABILITATION

Much of my clinical practice as an occupational therapist has been in the area of acute and post-acute TBI rehabilitation. Acute-care TBI rehabilitation focuses on medically stabilizing the individual and providing therapy to enhance physical and cognitive functions–for example, walking, speaking, feeding, and toileting. Post-acute care TBI rehabilitation promotes independent functioning in community living skills–such as, self-care, home management, meal preparation, and community travel.

In my clinical work in long-term, post-acute TBI rehabilitation, I observed that the preservation of life and the rehabilitation of physical and cognitive functions were not always personally meaningful to the individual if he or she could not also rebuild a quality of life worth maintaining. As an occupational therapist–trained to assist in the rehabilitation of primarily physical and cognitive skills–I began to feel ineffective and questioned the adequacy of a health care system able to preserve severely shattered bodies using advanced technology, but unable to help such individuals attain a personally satisfying quality of life after injury. It is my belief that while western medicine has become proficient in the care of acute medical crises, our health care system is ineffectual when dealing with long-term chronic disabilities and their resultant sequelae.

My clinical observation of males having long-term TBI (2+ years) suggested that many felt inadequately able to fulfill their personal adult male role expectations after injury. Many males expressed anger and sadness over their inability to marry, father children, achieve success in their chosen vocation, and participate in their communities as respected and valued community members.

While I observed this phenomenon with most of the adult males I treated in clinical practice, written accounts of post-TBI gender role strain were difficult to find in the TBI rehabilitation literature. Instead, several researchers of TBI rehabilitation documented the sexual disinhibition and socially inappropriate behavioral patterns that can sometimes accompany brain injury. Researchers also collected data regarding the long-term psychosocial sequelae of social isolation and the high divorce rate that tends to occur in marriages touched by the TBI of a partner. Literature was scant, however, that described the post-TBI male gender role strain that I and fellow therapists observed in practice. Still worse was the accompanying lack of treatment protocols designed to adequately resolve male gender role strain after TBI.

In response to this dearth of information regarding post-TBI gender role strain, I conducted a qualitative study that examined the impact of TBI on gender identity and role (Gutman & Napier-Klemic, 1996). Females were included in the study to determine how TBI influenced the perceptions of female participants' gender identity and role. The inclusion of females became an important aspect of this study, as much of my clinical practice dealt primarily with adult males. Because males sustain TBI four times as often as females, little research was available that explored the female experience of TBI. Research regarding women with TBI continues to be scarce to this date. Initially, I suspected that females, too, were likely experiencing a form of gender role strain similar to that which I observed in males.

This initial study queried the participants' about their experience of living with a TBI through six in-depth, open-ended interviews that occurred over a four-month period. Males described having lost most or all of the pre-injury social roles and relationships that enabled them to feel like adult males. At 2+ years post-injury males reported an inability to rebuild gender roles and to fulfill their expectations of an adult male lifestyle.

Women, conversely, reported that they did not lose many of the pre-injury roles and relationships that defined their identities as adult females. Female gender roles that were lost were either rebuilt post-injury or substituted by the adoption of similar roles that fulfilled personal expectations of being female. I was surprised to find that despite the adversity of sustaining a TBI, these women were able to create lives that were personally meaningful and facilitated continued growth as adult women. The finding that females tend to rebuild lost gender roles post-injury, while males experience a declining opportunity to engage in gender specific roles as length of time post-injury increases, was corroborated by several other researchers (Moore et al., 1994; Schmidt et al., 1995).

I wondered if males could learn to rebuild the gender social roles and activities that enable them to feel like adult men–much as females are socialized to do in western society. Based on this speculation, I developed a set of guidelines for practice designed to enhance male gender role satisfaction after TBI. This set of guidelines was founded on the premise that females do not commonly experience post-injury gender role strain primarily because they have learned–through a cultural socialization process–to build roles and to participate in activities that fulfill their personal experience of what it means to be female. I reasoned that if males with TBI could learn to rebuild the roles and activities that allowed the expression of male gender identity, post-TBI gender role strain could be alleviated.

In this book, I recount the story of four adult men who voluntarily participated in an occupational therapy intervention project in which they learned the skills to rebuild and maintain the adult male gender roles and activities they had either lost or never attained as a result of TBI. The following chapters are a journey through the men's learning experiences, setbacks, and personal growth.

Chapter 2

The Histories of Four Men with TBI

RUDY

Rudy, a childhood nickname for Rudolph, was the oldest of the four participants at 48 years of age. Rudy was an Italian-American, white, heterosexual male of thin build and average height. The large frame eyeglasses that sat crookedly across the bridge of his nose, magnified a deep facial scar that betrayed a past traumatic incident. At the age of 23, Rudy sustained a head injury in a motor vehicle accident (MVA) in which substance abuse was indicated. At the time of his injury, Rudy had just returned from Vietnam and was working as a longshoreman on the docks of a northeastern metropolitan city. The drug habit and heavy drinking pattern that was likely responsible for Rudy's accident had been developed during Rudy's military tour of duty in Vietnam.

Rudy grew up in an Italian-American family in which male and female roles were distinct and served to maintain traditional sex-based activities and patterns of interaction. He was the second born of two sons and described himself as having been competitive with his brother and "always coming up second best in school, the military, and with the ladies." Rudy expressed strong feelings of inadequacy in comparison to his brother, both before and after injury. He referred to his brother as the "good son" and verbalized that he wished he had developed into a man who, like his brother, had obtained a college degree, married, had children, and built a successful business. Instead,

[Haworth co-indexing entry note]: "The Histories of Four Men with TBI." Gutman, Sharon A. Co-published simultaneously in *Occupational Therapy in Mental Health* (The Haworth Press, Inc.) Vol. 15, No. 3/4, 2000, pp. 13-25; and: *Brain Injury and Gender Role Strain: Rebuilding Adult Lifestyles After Injury* (Sharon A. Gutman) The Haworth Press, Inc., 2000, pp. 13-25. Single or multiple copies of this article are available for a fee from The Haworth Document Delivery Service [1-800-342-9678, 9:00 a.m. - 5:00 p.m. (EST). E-mail address: getinfo@haworthpressinc.com].

13

Rudy perceived himself to be a burden and a disappointment to his family.

> I wish I had achieved what my brother has. And been in his [life] position. I'm a disappointment to Dad. I should be taking care of Dad right now in his elderly years, instead of him always helping me. I should be in the position to take Dad into my home. Instead, I'm a client at [facility's name] in a community group home with a bunch of guys with head injuries.

Rudy described himself as a "ladies' man" before injury and indicated that his greatest disappointment concerned his inability to form and sustain a committed relationship with a female. Although Rudy was married for two years between the ages of 40-42 he expressed that the marriage was personally unsatisfactory and believed that his ex-wife married him only for his insurance settlement. While Rudy reported being highly sexually active prior to his injury, he indicated that he lacked opportunities to engage in sexual activity with females post-injury.

> Finding women here [inside of the residential head injury facility] is like trying to find water in a desert. I used to date a lot. Now I feel like a penned up stag. What am I supposed to say to some lady I may meet outside of [facility's name]? Come over to my group home? Come hang out with the guys? I just want someone I can be loving with and who'd love me too. I haven't been touched by another human being in so long.

Rudy's pre-injury work role was highly meaningful to him and served to provide a strong male gender identity. He considered himself to be a workaholic and valued his ability to succeed in a traditional male gender role.

> Before my accident I was the man, boy. I worked the docks all night and into the wee hours of the morning. Two guys couldn't do what I got done. I wish I could find work like that now. Work that gave my life meaning like before. Not like the such and such jobs at the [facility's sheltered] workshop. Those jobs are so mindless they'd make you brain damaged if you weren't already.

Rudy was speaking of the facility's sheltered workshop where the residents would carry out unskilled jobs or piece work–packaging candy or breadsticks, sealing sponges in their plastic bag containers for mass sale, securing a specific number of brochures together with rubber bands, or packaging products in boxes. Large companies would bid out these jobs to the lowest charging sheltered workshop. While some residents appeared to enjoy their work, many looked forward most to the 10:00 a.m. coffee and cigarette break, lunch, and the 3:00 p.m. bell marking the end of the workday.

Rudy had chosen not to work since he did not find his vocational opportunities to be personally meaningful. After a couple of months at the facility's workshop Rudy refused to return. He was then offered a job raking leaves on the grounds of the facility and a neighboring child daycare program. While Rudy enjoyed seeing the children, he found this type of physical work to be drudgery and began to increasingly miss workdays due to backaches. Eventually Rudy refused to participate in any further work.

Prior to his injury, Rudy engaged in several activities that supported his role as an adult man. He reported that he could often be found in pool halls and dance clubs, and frequently attended live sporting events.

> I used to be out until morning, dancing, drinking, playing pool–just living life to the fullest. Now, it's a big night if I watch Late Night with Letterman.

According to one of the neuropsychologists who worked with him, Rudy began his current residence in the facility's residential head injury program four years ago. Initially, Rudy was admitted into the main campus facility but was quickly transferred to a shared community group home as a result of his cognitive ability to perform most self-care activities with distant supervision–including bathing, toileting, grooming, dressing, and basic household chores. However, due to his short-term memory deficits, Rudy continued to require close supervision for more complex activities of daily living–including meal preparation and money management. Although he also possessed the ability to remember the walking routes around his local community in order to independently access shopping, movies, recreational entertainment, and restaurants, Rudy required the accompaniment of a staff member in the larger community due to his impulsivity and tendency to be socially inappropriate in public–a facility decision that Rudy despised as it caused him to feel penalized for having a head injury.

SAL

Salvatore, known as Sal, was the second oldest of the four participants at 44 years of age. Sal, too, was an Italian-American, white, heterosexual male whose family of origin enacted traditional male and female roles. A tall, thin man who was seldom seen without a cigarette, Sal reported that he had sustained two brain injuries–the first occurred at 25 years of age in an alcohol-related motor vehicle accident in which Sal was determined to be driving while intoxicated (DWI). Sal's second TBI occurred at age 32, again, under similar circumstances of DWI.

Head injury, however, was not Sal's first experience with disability. As a child Sal contracted polio and was required to wear lower extremity braces for several years; Sal could not remember how many years. Like Rudy, Sal was the second born of two sons in an Italian-American family and experienced jealousy regarding what he perceived to be his older brother's greater competency and success in school, dating, athletics, and the military. Although Sal felt infantalized by his mother as a result of his childhood polio, he attempted to compensate for his disability in adolescence and early adulthood through high school athletics, pursuit of a college education, and entrance into the military.

His attempts to overcome his self-perceived inadequacies, however, fell short of his expectations and hopes. Sal was discharged from the military when his past medical history was uncovered. His childhood polio left him with a subtle but permanent vertebral and lower extremity orthopedic deformity that would have disqualified him from military entrance had he not lied about his medical history to enlist. As an ironic and cruel twist of fate, his discharge from the service coincided with his brother's promotion to an officer's status.

Instead of returning to college after his military discharge–which he left in order to enlist–Sal began a masonry and contracting business. He was invited to play lead and bass guitar in a cousin's band and quickly became enmeshed in the drug culture of the 1960s and early 70s. At that time, Sal married a 17 year old girlfriend whom he had been dating for just over one year. The marriage was precipitated by a pregnancy that later ended in a miscarriage. For the next three years Sal successfully supported himself and his wife through his masonry and contracting work but became more heavily involved with drugs and alcohol. At age 25, Sal sustained his first severe head injury and began a five-year residential rehabilitation process on the west coast. It is likely that Sal was transferred to the west coast for TBI rehabilitation due to the lack of facilities specializing in brain injury care at that time–the late 1970s.

At the end of his first rehabilitation period, Sal returned home to the northeast to find that his wife had obtained a divorce from him and, having no job prospects or adequate community living skills, he was forced to move into his mother's house. Sal remembers this as a period of hopelessness.

> Mother didn't want me home. But she accepted my money anyway. I felt unwanted. You know, a burden. She treated me like a helpless infant. I'd get high just to deal with her and the awfulness of the situation.

During the first year that he was living in his mother's house, Sal frequented bars, freely obtained drugs from friends, and commonly utilized the services of prostitutes. He met a prostitute who accepted his proposal of marriage and both moved into an apartment together. The marriage was characterized by heavy drinking and fighting. Several months later, Sal literally crawled back to his mother's house and begged to be taken in. He had a host of cuts and bruises on his body that he said had occurred in the habitual physical frays he had with his wife. Sal's mother helped him obtain a divorce and agreed that he could move back into her home as long as he remained sober. Shortly after Sal returned to his mother's home at the age of 32, he sustained his second TBI in another alcohol-related motor vehicle accident. It was unclear whether Sal was even licensed to drive at this time, although it is likely that he was not, as he reported that he had been taking medication for a seizure disorder resulting from his first TBI. After sustaining his second TBI in his mother's old '72 Chevy Malibu, Sal began yet another five-year residential rehabilitation process at the same west coast facility where he spent five years recovering from his first TBI.

When Sal's insurance funding finally dissipated, he was then returned to his mother–who could now no longer physically care for him. At this time, Sal began his current residential placement in the community group home program. Upon admission into the group home program, Sal excelled with minimal to moderate supervision from staff members. At first Sal was well liked by staff–as he was polite in an old-fashioned gentlemanly way and caused little disruption in the day-to-day routine of the community group home into which he was placed. Sal was quite and remained alone most of the time. It was rare that he asked the group home staff members to help him with any task, instead performing most daily living activities independently. According to one staff member, Sal was considered to be so independent that several staff members questioned why he even required group home living. After several months, and the recommendation of Sal's treatment team, he was transferred from the group home to a dual-occupancy apartment with another male client. Here in the apartment program, Sal received 12 hours of distant supervision as opposed to the 24 hours of on-sight supervision provided in the group home program. The 12 hours of supervision were divided as such: 4-6 hours of actual contact with the client throughout the day and evening, and 6-8 hours of contact via phone access. With only 12 hours of distant supervision from staff, Sal began to experience past difficulties. On two separate occasions, drugs were found in his possession. And after a safety incident in which Sal ignited a fire by leaving a cigarette burning, he was moved back to the community group home program. This was viewed by Sal as a demotion and personal failure.

> I feel bad that I was sent back to the group home from the apartments. I don't want to see the friends I made there. They look down upon me now because I'm not as smart or competent as them–I can't live in the apartments like them. That's what they think, that I need to be *supervised* [Sal says this word with sarcasm and anger in his voice].

Sal was fully ambulatory and had achieved independent travel status in the community. Although Sal exhibited severe short-term memory difficulties, he was able to function in activities of daily living with the assistance of a memory/schedule book. He was also able to maintain a volunteer position at a local nursing home in which he transported nonambulatory wheelchair-bound patients to different therapies within the facility. Sal found this work to be personally meaningful and rewarding.

> My job at [name of nursing home] is important to me. I feel like I'm doing something to help others–taking the seniors to their therapies. It makes me feel like I can do a valuable thing for other

people. And it's a place where I feel appreciated. The seniors–the ones who can remember me–are glad to see me. They just want to have someone who's nice to them and who will listen. Just like anybody who feels alone.

ED

Ed was a 30 year old Irish-American, white, heterosexual male who, at the age of 21, sustained a head injury after falling asleep at the wheel of his delivery truck one Monday morning after a sleep deprived weekend of overtime work and late night televised ball games. Ed's ability to read and interpret social cues was perhaps the most impaired of the four men described in this book, and most likely reflected the existence of poor pre-injury social skills. Ed conjured up the appearance of a child in a man's body–an unsophisticated, unsuspecting, trustful child who wants only to please others and be praised. As a result of his neurologic injury, Ed walked with a wide-based gait pattern similar to the developmental stage of a two-year old who has not gained precision control and coordinated sequencing of his limbs. His speech had become dysarthric (slurred) and difficult to understand as a result of injury, and further added to the illusion of childlike innocence. Ed's facial expressions and body language, too, readily reflected the direct eagerness, enthusiasm, and anger of a child who has not learned to modulate his emotions. Nothing betrayed his adult age outside of his 5'10", 200 lb. body frame, his facial hair, the lines and crevices across his forehead and face, and the deepness of his voice when raised in anger.

Prior to his accident, Ed had finished high school and was working full-time as a delivery person for a local tire company. He had been steadily dating a female friend whom he met in high school; however, the relationship was not physical and appeared more to resemble the buddy-type relationships that Ed maintained with his male friends. Ed had also remained friends with two childhood male buddies who lived on the same neighborhood street and grew up with Ed. These were the friends who comprised Ed's social circle–a group of good boys from working-class families, who grew up in the Boy Scouts and neither excelled in sports, academics, nor rebelliousness. They spent their school nights and weekends bowling in a neighborhood league, attending ball games at school and in the city, and working part-time jobs: delivering newspapers, shoveling snow, cutting grass, and pumping gas. They were unnoticed, neither excelling nor causing trouble in their families, schools, and communities.

At the time of his accident, Ed was living at home with his parents and younger siblings. Ed grew up in a large Irish-American family located in a northeastern urban city. His biological father had reportedly died prior to Ed's birth. When Ed's mother remarried, her new husband agreed to adopt and raise Ed as his own son. The couple then produced four sons in addition to Ed. Ed did not learn that his father was not his biological parent until the age of 16, but he described growing up with a distinct feeling that his father favored his four younger brothers.

> My father didn't have much to do with me. He'd spend a lot of time with my brothers but not me. I never knew why. I thought there musta been something wrong with me. I didn't know that my real father died until I was 16. I was shocked–I'm still shocked. The only thing I got from him [biological father] was his [first] name, Edmund.

It is unfortunate that Ed describes being unable to develop close bonds with his brothers–who may have unconsciously perceived their father's cues and further ostracized Ed.

> My brothers and I weren't close growing up. They did their own things. They played softball with my Dad but not me. I always thought it was because I couldn't hit as well as them. I felt bad for them, having a big brother who couldn't teach em how to hit a baseball. Anyway, they're all married now. They have their own lives and I don't bother 'em.

The discussion of other people's marriages, children, jobs, and homes littered Ed's speech. It appeared that he had not only internalized, but embraced his culture's value of marriage, parenting, work, and home ownership as indicators of an adult status. Ed appeared particularly concerned that he had not achieved these adult roles while his younger brothers had.

> I'm the oldest son. I should have been married first. My brothers all have wives and kids and their own homes. Every night I

wonder when it's gonna happen to me. I pray every night for God to help me be the man I always thought I'd be. I won't give up cause I know God is listening.

Following Ed's accident and one year rehabilitation period, he moved into his parents' home for several months. His parents, however, could neither physically care for Ed nor emotionally understand his altered personality and sought placement for him in a residential head injury facility. The good boy that they raised now had unpredictable mood swings, bursts of anger caused from frustration, and a tendency to neglect his personal hygiene. Ed's parents thought about the effect that Ed would have on the two youngest sons who were still living at home. They decided that it would be best for everyone if Ed moved to a residential rehabilitation facility that specialized in brain injury. Ed has lived in this facility for the last five years.

When I met Ed, he resided in a community group home housing four other males with TBI. He worked four 5 hour days in a sheltered workshop where he assembled packages of office supplies, advertisement brochures, candy, toys, and household cleaning products. On some days Ed performed custodial duties in the workshop, cleaning the floors and emptying the trash. He took great pride in the performance of his work and seemed to glow in the praise bestowed by his supervisors. Ed was thought of as a good client at the facility, never causing the staff members any concern. He had mastered the skill of fitting in by doing everything right, long ago.

In the community group home where Ed lived, he performed the self-care activities of bathing, grooming, and dressing independently, and always finished his chores of laundry, cleaning, and vacuuming without being asked. He consistently maintained the cleanliness and neatness of his own room as though he was expecting guests any minute. In the community, Ed required close supervision with more complex activities of daily living (ADL) such as meal preparation, shopping, banking, money management, and community travel. If in adolescence Ed was the good Boy Scout who could be counted on to carry the Boy Scout Manual when everyone else had lost theirs, in adulthood Ed had become the good client who could be counted on to remain quiet and polite when everyone else was in the midst of a "behavioral incident."

JAY

Jay, the youngest of the four men at 27 years of age, was a white, heterosexual male of Russian-Jewish descent. Although Jay's slight body frame heightened his youthful appearance, his staccato voice and need for a cane during ambulation gave him the illusion of old age–a personal trait that was not entirely incongruent with an apparent wisdom beyond his years. When Jay was a 19 year old college sophomore, he sustained a head injury in a motor vehicle accident caused by a freak mechanical error. The tire rim of his front car wheel blew off causing Jay to lose control of his car.

Like the other three men, Jay's childhood and adolescence were marked by difficulty and struggle. As a child, Jay was diagnosed with obsessive compulsive disorder (OCD) and attention-deficit-hyperactivity disorder (ADHD). Jay describes himself as having been a difficult child to raise.

> I was a handful to my parents. I was always into something I wasn't supposed to be. The neighbors hated me. They [his parents] sent me to boarding school because, I don't know, I guess they couldn't have me in the house or live with me or something. It wasn't a normal childhood, you know, like kids living with their parents. I felt very alone most of the time. I never really felt like I had a real family.

Like Ed, Jay did not grow up with his biological father. His mother and biological father divorced when Jay was four. Jay's mother remarried a man who, again like Ed, agreed to raise Jay as his own son. But a child with OCD and ADHD may have been difficult for Jay's stepfather to accept. Jay remembers being yelled at and slapped by his stepfather.

> My stepfather coached my little league. I was really good. I was better than any other kid–I was that good. But if I did something wrong or fooled around my stepfather would punch me hard in the gut or yell at me all the time. I was always getting yelled at, it seems, no matter what I did or how hard I tried to act like he wanted me to. And then I think I just stopped trying. I basically said, "up yours," to my stepfather and stopped playing sports.

After Jay's mother and stepfather married they had two daughters. Jay reported fighting heavily with both girls throughout childhood.

The second-born daughter, who was 10 years younger than Jay, was physically too small to defend herself and Jay believed that his parents sent him to boarding school to preserve a modicum of family peace. Jay remembers this period as a time of loneliness.

> I didn't like boarding school–what I can remember of it. I wanted to be a normal kid and live at home with my parents. I didn't have any friends there. I guess I mostly hung out by myself. Like always.

The behaviors that Jay exhibited as a result of having OCD and ADHD made it difficult for him to maintain friendships while growing up. Jay reported never having formed any close friends in childhood or adolescence.

> I never really had any friends. It's not that I didn't want friends. People thought I was weird, I guess, and didn't wanna have much to do with me. Like I'd be touching things over and over again. It's part of the OCD; I have to touch certain objects repeatedly to make them clean. And the other kids would call me freaky and other mean stuff. But you know, now I understand that they acted that way cause they didn't understand and I was different. And it's an unfortunate part of human nature to ridicule and ostracize what's different from you.

Jay's preoccupation with the positioning of items and his need to repeat purposeless actions were still apparent in his adult behaviors. It was difficult for Jay to leave a room without repeatedly checking to see that he had closed the door tightly or returned a chair precisely to its original grooves in the carpet.

Although Jay reported that he did not have many friends as a child and adolescent, he nevertheless participated in a number of group sports including softball, ping pong, swimming, and track.

> The ironic thing was that I excelled at sports or any kinda activity where I could indulge my [physical] speed and obsessions. Like pin pong–that was really a sport where I could let my OCD fly. Hitting the ball with my paddle over and over was an obsessive's delight. I'd think in my head, "I have to touch the ball with my paddle 50 times without missing," or I'd have to start counting all over again. Or in the pool I'd have to count how many strokes

> it would take to get from one end of the pool to the other. These were things I did that nobody knew. No one knew I was obsessively counting my strokes–they just saw me as a good swimmer. I liked playing sports with other guys. It was a way I could be around them without feeling like I was really different and weird. I was really good, too, [at sports] so they liked to have me on their teams.

Additionally, Jay considered himself to be a self-taught musician having learned both piano and acoustic guitar independently.

At the time of Jay's TBI, he had been living away from home and attending a college in the northeast. While he reported that he continued to lack friendships, he had developed a dating relationship with a female college student of his own age. This female was sitting in the passenger side of the vehicle in which Jay's accident occurred. Unlike Jay, she walked away from the accident unscathed. Although his memory of the events that occurred around the time of his accident is hazy, Jay could not remember having contact with his girlfriend after recovering consciousness in the hospital.

Jay's biological father, who had failed to be a consistent presence in Jay's childhood, completely severed contact with him after his accident. His biological father's abandonment and his poor relationship with his stepfather left Jay without positive male role models and mentors in childhood, adolescence, and early adulthood.

At the time of the study, Jay had been attending the facility's community group home program for two years. He reported having no friends in the facility and said that he often inadvertently angered other clients without understanding why. Jay no longer displayed the hyperactivity apparent in childhood; as a result of his head injury, the part of Jay's brain that regulates alertness became impaired, causing him to easily experience fatigue with little exertion.

Unfortunately, Jay's TBI exacerbated his pre-morbid tendency to display distractibility and inattention. His inability to focus on a task for more than five minutes at a time had hindered his ability to obtain greater independence in community living skills. According to Jay's rehabilitation case manager, Jay required close supervision to perform self-care activities–such as, grooming, bathing, and dressing–and complex ADLs requiring the ability to maintain attention for a length of time–meal preparation, money management, shopping, and community travel. Despite Jay's concentration difficulties, he nevertheless displayed a very high level of intelligence, extreme quick wit, and considerable creativity–skills that were readily apparent in his conversations.

While Jay was perhaps the most intellectually gifted of the four men, he was also the most physically challenged. As a result of his neurologic impairment, Jay displayed upper and lower extremity hemiparesis (weakness) and a left visual hemianopsia (field cut). At the time of the intervention, Jay had just begun to walk with a straight cane for short distances, after several years of wheelchair ambulation. Prior to Jay's admission to his present community group home program he had lived in another TBI residential facility where his physical status had been neglected. Jay's ability to walk had decreased as a result of disuse, as it was easier for staff to leave him in a wheelchair than to spend the time needed to exercise his lower extremities.

Chapter 3

The Men's Experience
of Gender Role Strain After TBI

In the previous chapters, gender role strain was defined as a feeling of uncertainty regarding one's ability to participate in the desired roles of adulthood after the onset of disability–particularly roles that allow the expression of one's gender identity. Gender is the perception of oneself as a male or female. The concept of gender is believed to develop in early childhood when children begin to think of themselves as girls or boys. Traditionally, in western culture there have been specific social roles identified as male or female. In recent years, sex-specific social roles have become blurred as females have assumed gender roles that have been traditionally defined as masculine–for example, the worker role and the bread-winner. However, while greater opportunities to assume male gender roles have been available to women, the same has not been true for males. Men, largely, have not assumed what has been traditionally thought of as female gender social roles. This may account for why a greater number of males tend to report gender role strain after TBI–there are less socially acceptable roles in the culture that allow men to express their male gender identity (Lindsey, 1994).

In this book, the concept of male gender role strain is used to describe the experience of men who perceive their internal personality traits to be congruent with their personal expectations of masculinity,

[Haworth co-indexing entry note]: "The Men's Experience of Gender Role Strain After TBI." Gutman, Sharon A. Co-published simultaneously in *Occupational Therapy in Mental Health* (The Haworth Press, Inc.) Vol. 15, No. 3/4, 2000, pp. 27-47; and: *Brain Injury and Gender Role Strain: Rebuilding Adult Lifestyles After Injury* (Sharon A. Gutman) The Haworth Press, Inc., 2000, pp. 27-47. Single or multiple copies of this article are available for a fee from The Haworth Document Delivery Service [1-800-342-9678, 9:00 a.m. - 5:00 p.m. (EST). E-mail address: getinfo@haworthpressinc.com].

but who–as a result of traumatic disability–feel denied access to male roles in the larger society. Males with TBI who used pre-injury masculine gender roles and activities to express their masculine gender identity, commonly report post-injury gender role strain if they are unable to engage in those roles and activities after the onset of their disability. Such males express frustration regarding their unsuccessful attempts to achieve self-perceived masculine adult roles after disability (e.g., worker, economic provider, husband/sexual partner, father). Often, as length of time post-injury increases, participation in masculine gender social roles and activities decreases. Males with TBI frequently become socially isolated after injury, refrain from participation in pre-injury male gender roles and activities, and fail to rebuild pre-injury relationships that support a male gender identity.

As mentioned previously, males with TBI report greater gender role strain than do females. Because western males may be culturally socialized to refrain from help-seeking in crisis, they may be more susceptible than females to social isolation and gender role strain post-TBI. Males may also believe that participation in traditionally masculine gender roles alone can provide a sense of gender role satisfaction, and thus fail to engage in post-injury gender-neutral social roles and activities that may provide adequate masculine role expression.

In this chapter, the four men's experience of gender role strain after TBI is examined. Typically, men who have sustained some type of traumatic disability experience gender role strain in three primary life areas: (a) the participation in male gender social roles, (b) the participation in male gender activities, and (c) the transition through rites of passage into male adulthood. Male gender social roles are the societal positions that indicate the assumption of male adulthood. Male gender activities are the occupations, avocations, and daily life projects that support a man's ability to assume a particular male gender role. Male gender rites of passage are the life events that mark the transition from male adolescence to adulthood. Males who sustain TBI commonly lose their pre-injury male gender roles, activities, and relationships, and find that they are unable to rebuild a post-injury lifestyle that is congruent with their perceptions of male adulthood. After injury, Rudy, Sal, Ed, and Jay found that they were unable to construct lifestyles that met their own expectations of what it means to be an adult man.

PARTICIPATION IN MALE GENDER SOCIAL ROLES

It is important to note that each of the four men had not equally assumed the roles characteristic of male adulthood prior to injury. Among the four men a range existed regarding the degree to which each had transitioned from adolescent to adult male gender roles. For example, Sal–the oldest of the four men to receive his injury–had firmly established participation in several adult male gender social roles while Jay–the youngest to sustain TBI–continued to occupy roles characteristic of adolescence.

By the time Sal experienced his first TBI at the age of 25, he had successfully developed his own masonry/contracting business, had married and become a homeowner, and was competently earning a salary sufficient to support himself and his wife. Rudy had also successfully transitioned into several roles of male adulthood. At 23 years of age–the time of his injury–Rudy was a Vietnam War Veteran who was earning a living as a longshoreman. This work enabled Rudy to independently support himself and maintain an apartment in a large urban city. Rudy had also established an active role in dating and sexual relationships with women and was seeking a committed relationship as a precursor to marriage.

Conversely, Ed was in the initial stages of transitioning from adolescent to adult roles when his injury occurred (at 21 years of age). At the time of his TBI, Ed had just begun to establish an adult work history, securing his first full-time job (as a driver/delivery person) just one year prior to injury. However, Ed had neither moved out of the parental home, nor developed the monetary management skills necessary to live independently in the community. Additionally, Ed had not established a role in dating relationships despite his strong interest in eventually securing a committed relationship with a female. While he spent considerable time with a female friend in high school, this relationship remained platonic and did not afford Ed the opportunity to learn courtship skills.

Unlike the other three men, Jay had not transitioned into roles characteristic of male adulthood prior to injury. Jay, who was a 19 year old college sophomore at the time of his injury, was the only one of the four men who was formally considered an adolescent when his injury occurred. At 19 years of age–on the threshold of transitioning from adolescent to adult roles–Jay had neither established an adult work history nor developed the skills necessary to live independently in the community. In fact, similar to Ed, Jay had never been required to support himself independently–transferring from the protective environment of the college dormitory to a rehabilitation facility offering supportive living arrangements. Like Ed, Jay did not develop courtship skills. Although, he had met and developed a relationship with a female prior to injury, the relationship was short-lived and did not afford Jay sufficient opportunity to learn the social interaction skills necessary to form and sustain dating relationships.

Loss of Pre-Injury Roles

The male gender social roles that the four men had constructed prior to injury can be seen in Table 3.1. These roles consisted of a variety of community member, friend, family, and dating/courtship roles. Each of the four men lost more than one-half of these pre-injury roles after TBI and could not rebuild them post-injury. Sal's loss of pre-injury male gender roles, and his inability to rebuild them after injury, was characteristic of the four men's experience.

> I was married and I was a property owner. I achieved all the things people have as life goals. After my first accident my marriage fell apart and she [Sal's wife] got a divorce from me. Wife two was no better. And every lady I meet now, she doesn't want to be with someone disabled. Or if it's a [name of rehabilitation facility] client, the staff won't let her out on a date. I haven't been in a relationship since my second accident.

Sal also lost his role as an independent home maintainer in the community.

> I built my own home before my accident. I even built my brother a house. But after my accident I've been back and forth between Mother's [home] and different rehab centers. And at [name of rehabilitation center], when they let me live in the apartments [shared apartment living in the community] they said I was a safety hazard and sent me back to the group home.

Prior to his first injury Sal had established the adult roles of husband, self-employed worker, and property owner. These roles afforded Sal the opportunity to participate in activities and relationships that

TABLE 3.1. Pre- and Post-Injury Roles and Activities

	Pre-Injury Roles	Post-Injury Roles	Pre-Injury Activities	Post-Injury Activities
SAL	• Husband • Brother • Son • Uncle • Friend • Self-Employed Worker • Musician • Sports Participant	• Volunteer • Client in TBI Facility • Community Group Home Member	• Built & Restored Homes & Furniture • Bought & Restored Sports Cars • Played Violin, Piano, Bass Guitar • Cooked Italian Cuisine • Played Pool & Cards • Used Alcohol & Drugs for Recreation	• Volunteered as a Client Transport in Nursing Home • Dined Alone in Community Restaurants • Maintained Personal Room in Group Home • Walked Around Neighbor-hood Alone • Followed Medication Routine • Exercised to Decrease Chronic Pain
RUDY	• Son • Brother • Friend • Worker • Independent Home Maintainer • Dating/Court-ship Participant • War Veteran • Sports Participant	• Client in TBI Facility • Community Group Home Member	• Dined with Female Companions • Engaged in Sexual Relationships • Attended Movies & Musicals • Played Pool & Cards • Patronized Bars & Dance Clubs • Used Alcohol & Drugs as Recreation • Unloaded Dock Ships	• Maintained Personal Room in Group Home • Completed Chores in Group Home • Slept 2-3 Hours per Day • Watched TV at Night • Perused Personal Ads • Followed Medication Routine
ED	• Son • Friend • Beginning Role in Dating/Court-ship • Sports Participant • Church Member	• Worker in Sheltered Workshop • Church Member	• Played High School Football • Attended Sporting Events • Bowled with a League • Sang in Church Choir	• Maintained personal Room in Group Home • Watched TV Alone in Room • Bowled Once per Month

TABLE 3.1 (continued)

	Pre-Injury Roles	Post-Injury Roles	Pre-Injury Activities	Post-Injury Activities
ED			• Worked in Pizza Shop	• Regular Weekly Church Attendance • Followed Medication Routine • Performed Self-Range of Motion Exercises
JAY	• Student • Son • Brother • Athlete • Musician • Beginning Role in Dating/Court-ship	• Client in TBI Facility • Community Group Home Member • Worker in Sheltered Workshop	• Attended College • Engaged in Creative Writing • Biked, Ran Track, Played Softball • Worked as Lifeguard • Played Piano • Played Pool & Ping-Pong	• Maintained Personal Room in Group Home • Completed Assigned Chores in Group Home • Attended Therapies (PT, Speech) • Followed Medication Routine • Performed Self-Range of Motion Exercises • Performed Orthotic Maintenance

allowed the expression of his male gender identity. After his first injury, Sal lost these roles and was unable to rebuild them. Even when Sal appeared to make progress toward the resumption of a role–such as remarrying after injury or advancing to the community apartment program–his attempts were unsuccessful and he was left feeling less competent to participate in adult male roles.

Feelings of Abandonment and Victimization

The four men also lost important relationships that accompanied their pre-injury gender social roles. Themes of abandonment and estrangement after injury pervaded their stories. Sal reported having a close relationship with his father until his first TBI, at which time his father grew more distant and died shortly after as a result of a heart attack.

> My dad was someone I could talk to about anything. I considered him my closest friend. After my accident he [father] stayed longer and longer hours at work. We never talked about my head injury. Nothing about how it affected all of our lives. And then he died when I was away at the rehab in California.

For Sal, the death of his father not only meant the loss of a trusted confidant but also the loss of the family member who was able to buffer the conflicted relationship Sal shared with his mother.

> After Dad died, Mother became more and more controlling. I felt she was resentful at having me in her house. She made me feel unwanted, like she was tired of having to take care of her little boy who should have grown up a long time ago.

Jay, too, reported feelings of estrangement from his family.

> I feel pushed out of my family. I'm scared that the distance will develop between me and my mom as it was years ago when they [parents] sent me to boarding school. I don't feel real close to my mom. I love her. I think she's tried to be helpful, but I feel distanced from her.

> My stepfather has been polite to me since my accident but we don't really have a relationship. It's been so many years of distance where we haven't been father and son. I don't feel that I know him at all. . . . I don't see my sisters much either. I don't really know them well. . . . I don't feel good about being a son. I don't feel close to my parents or my sisters really.

> My father remarried and had other children [when Jay was a child]. They [father and stepsiblings] don't come to see me now. My real father excommunicated me after my accident. I feel real bad about that. I wish I had a life that was normal.

Feelings of abandonment for these men also stemmed from significant others and friends.

When I had my accident and I was in the hospital, I couldn't talk or walk. I'd just make noises like this [verbally utters unintelligible sounds]. [Girlfriend's name] came to see me once and she saw I couldn't walk or talk and she never came back. She forgot about me. I tried to call her a couple of times but she didn't call me back. (Ed)

I tried to call my girlfriend a couple of times after my injury, but she never kept in touch. Basically, I guess you can say that she went on with her life. I got the feeling that she was uncomfortable around me. Maybe I reminded her of what coulda happened to her. (Jay)

I did a lot of free work for my friends–building decks and additions, fixin up their old junk houses they thought was so valuable. Now they're not around when I need them. It's like being discarded. Dropped when you ain't needed no more. (Sal)

For some of the men, feelings of abandonment and estrangement after injury were accompanied by deep anger and resentment. The theme of feeling betrayed and victimized by formally trusted loved ones and friends–whom the men had helped in times of past crisis–weighed heavily on their sense of outrage. Below, Sal articulately conveyed his anger toward his family members for betraying his trust at a time when he was dependent upon their care.

My role as my mother's son has not been personally satisfying for years. She was taking my finances while I was in the hospital and paying her mortgage with it. I couldn't trust her. Her name was on my accounts because of my accident. One of my therapists helped me to see a lawyer to remove her as my guardian. Now Mother and I have very little to say. I don't feel like a son to my mother anymore.

I built my brother a house [before Sal's accident]. He sold it when he divorced. Now he's living in the house I owned for ten years. Mother took it when she became my legal guardian. I feel very bitter about this. She was making money off of renting my house while I was in the hospital. Then she gave it to my brother and his wife. I feel very resentful. I try not to think about it. I don't speak to my brother anymore.

When I was in the hospital the first time, my wife was cheating on me and got a divorce from me. And wife two completely used me for my money [insurance settlement].

Rudy also mirrored Sal's sentiments of betrayal and outrage.

That crazy bat [wife] used me for my insurance settlement. I didn't see what was what until I had said "I do." Despite my family's protests. After two years and ten thousand dollars later, now I know better–the hard way.

The Deterioration of an Adult Male Identity After Injury

Additionally, new roles that each of the four men assumed post-injury neither preserved pre-injury relationships nor encouraged the expression of male gender identity. As seen in Table 3.1, the major roles that the participants assumed post-injury were those of a client in a TBI rehabilitation facility and a community group home member. The men reported that these roles served to further deteriorate their identities as adult men.

I don't feel like I'm an adult here, or looked upon as an adult here [in the TBI rehabilitation facility]. I'm treated like an adolescent, what with all the assigned chores and the [weekly monetary] allowances. And the dating opportunities. Oh boy, [name of facility] is just a swinging singles club. Maybe if I lived in the apartments I'd have more privacy–I could invite a lady over for dinner. But not here in the group home–in the cub scout's house. I just don't feel like I'm given the chances to act like an adult. (Rudy)

Being a client with a head injury is a career in itself. And being a client makes your gender neutral. It's like you lose what it's like to be a man. (Rudy)

Isolation After Injury

Roles established post-injury often facilitated isolation. For example, while Ed was able to rebuild his role as a church participant, his regular Sunday attendance did not help him to forge relationships with others. In fact, the church that Ed attended attempted to accommodate individuals with disabilities by providing a special pew directly in front of the congregation for easy accessibility. However, while the church's accommodation was meant with good intent, setting Ed aside from the church congregation did not help him to meet and establish friendships with other church members.

Dissatisfaction with Their Inability to Meet Personal Male Role Expectations

All of the men expressed dissatisfaction with their ability to meet personal male role expectations after injury.

> A part of my life is missing. It's like living somebody else's life. I know it's me. But it just doesn't seem like me–I mean like the me I thought I'd be as an adult man. It's like after the accident happened they mixed up the bodies and I got put back together in someone else's life. Like a movie. I keep thinking, "Don't you [other people] realize this isn't me? This is not the kind of lifestyle I was supposed to have. Hey, who's in charge here? Someone made a big mistake!" (Rudy)

> I'm not the adult I could have been if things were different, if the accident had never happened. My life would be totally different. I would be a totally different person with a totally different lifestyle. (Jay)

> I haven't met the expectations I had for myself. I might have met them for a short time previously–before my accident–but no more. Each day is a reminder of what I lost and can't seem to get back. After awhile you just give up trying. It's like you're in the twilight zone and nobody realizes it but you. And in the beginning you do anything to get back your real self. But no one seems to listen or help. And after lots of time goes by you start believing that the twilight zone is normal. (Sal)

Specifically, the men expressed disappointment regarding their inability to assume the roles of spouse, father, worker, independent home maintainer, and friend.

This house I'm living in here at [name of facility], this is the kind of house I thought I'd live in with my wife and kids. Not as a group home member with a head injury. That really hits me where I live. I just think that if I hadn't had this head injury I would have been married with a kid or two and living in a house like this one. The irony kills me. (Rudy)

I've wanted a relationship for years now. I want a wife and family of my own. All of my brothers are married. I keep asking, "When's it gonna be me?" When will it be my turn? (Ed)

Once or twice I saw a bus with school children and it really tugged at my heart, that I don't have any children of my own. You know, I never thought about kids because I always just assumed that I'd get married and the little ones would come in time. It's amazing the things you take for granted. (Rudy)

I had a good job before my accident. I didn't want to give it up. Cause I really worked hard to get a job. I used to cry a lot about losing the job; it was something I worked real hard for. It felt like a defeat to me. (Ed)

I miss the male camaraderie I used to have before my injury. Just shoot'n the breeze with the guys. It used to make me feel like I belonged. Men are like animals; they run in packs. You know, that male bonding thing–it hasn't happened here [at the rehabilitation facility]. I don't have too many friends here. It's like an oil and water thing I guess; I just don't know why I haven't been able to connect with anyone. (Rudy)

I'm not sure if I have friends now, I mean friends I'd really call true friends. I think I have sympathy friends–people who act like my friends because they feel sorry for me. (Jay)

I want my own apartment. I never lived alone like an adult. I went from living with my mother to living here [in a TBI rehabilitation facility]. I want to get to the apartments and live by myself. My younger brothers live on their own. I want to be independent too. I'm 30. I'm ready. I'm overdue. (Ed)

The men's reactions reflect feelings of derealization–"This can't be my life"–disappointment, depression, and denial. It is as though they have voiced an internal soliloquy that demanded to be vocalized.

Dissatisfaction with Their Inability to Meet Parental Expectations

Many of the men also expressed disappointment that they had not lived up to parental expectations of male role enactment.

> I know my dad would have wanted me to lead a different life. Have the wife and kids and a good job and a nice house where he could visit the grandkids. I know I'm a disappointment to him. I feel real bad about that. (Rudy)

> I guess my mother and stepdad expected me to get married and have a family. I guess that's what they wanted for me, what they thought would provide a happy life for me. But I don't think that I ever met their expectations before my accident and I guess I'm not meeting them now. Sometimes it's hard for me to deal with the feeling that I haven't measured up. But I'm trying my best. (Jay)

Moreover, several of the men expressed their belief that they had become a burden to their families by forcing family members to assume caregiver roles.

> It's been hard, if not harder on my family. That tears me apart. I feel like a burden to them. I wish I could change that. I really want my dad to see me a little more stable and competent–more like the man I know I can be–before he passes away. (Rudy)

> I don't want my dad to worry about me in his senior years–the years he should be living without a care in the world. You know, he's got his own health problems–his heart condition and etceteras. I shouldn't be adding to his worries. Being a man to me means not being a burden on my family. (Rudy)

> I don't want my mom and stepdad to feel burdened with my care the rest of their lives. As an adult I'd like to be self-supporting. After all that's what it means to be an adult–to be able to take care of yourself. (Jay)

Without the opportunity to express their feelings of regret and appreciation to family members, the men's emotions became suppressed demons waiting to come alive through nightmares and daytime panic attacks.

PARTICIPATION IN MALE GENDER ACTIVITIES

As seen in Table 3.1, the four men participated in an array of pre-injury activities that allowed the expression of their male gender identities–including engaging in and attending sporting events, buying and restoring sports cars, and dining out with female companions. Each of the men lost the ability to participate in more than one-half of these activities after injury and could not re-establish post-injury participation. The men were also unable to establish participation in new post-injury activities that could support the resumption of male gender roles. Predominant activities engaged in after injury included completing community group home assigned chores, maintaining one's personal room in the community group home, and attending to one's health maintenance secondary to TBI–for instance donning molded ankle-foot orthoses to increase ambulation ability, practicing self-range of motion exercises to reduce the likelihood of contractures, and adhering to a specific medication routine. These activities neither preserved participation in pre-injury male gender roles nor supported the acquisition of new post-injury male roles.

Participation in Adolescent Activities

Additionally, there appeared to be little opportunity in the environment for these men to participate in the activities of male adulthood; rather the activities that were readily available in the environment were more characteristic of adolescence and heightened the men's feelings of decreased daily life control. All of the men–except for Sal–received a weekly allowance from which they could budget their expenses. They were not permitted to deviate from a facility established routine designating specific times for work, chores, meals, and recreation. Often recreational opportunities consisted of watching rented videos–that someone else chose–in a community group home or going out to dinner with other group home members and staff. The men reported having little opportunity to engage in self-chosen activities or to chose with whom to spend time. In fact, engaging in isolative activities may have been one way in which the men exerted volitional choice–by spending time alone they were able to elect not to interact with other group home members who were assigned to share their residence, mealtimes, and recreational opportunities. Jay explained his lack of ability to exert his personal choice and independence:

> I don't feel particularly autonomous living here in a community group home. It's kind of like being a freshman in college forever. You don't choose where to live or who to live with. You're assigned your classes–but here [rehabilitation facility] it's your therapies. You have specific mealtimes and you can't choose what to eat.

Sal also experienced distress regarding his lack of ability to engage in self-chosen activities.

> That's why I like dining out by myself. I get to pick my own meal times and my own food preferences and I can have adult conversations and interact with the restaurant employees instead of trying to start up a conversation with the guys in the house [community group home]. Just because I live with them doesn't mean I gotta do other activities with them too. I have nothing in common with them other than the head injury.

Post-Injury Isolation and Inactivity

Post-injury participation in activities that facilitated social isolation was common among the four men. Listening to music and watching television alone in one's room were reported as frequently engaged in post-injury activities. Sal, who was officially cleared to walk around the community independently by his TBI rehabilitation team, commonly spent several hours walking the blocks of his neighborhood or dining out alone. While these activities may have afforded the men the privacy and volitional choice they felt they lacked, such isolative activities also failed to provide the opportunity to build post-injury relationships through which to engage in male gender roles.

Additionally, the men did not possess a daily repertoire of gender activities sufficient to occupy at least half of their day. Consequently, each man spent between two to three hours per day without activity. Sleeping and watching television were commonly used to fill hours as a result of decreased opportunities to participate in activities that could support the acquisition of post-injury male gender roles.

Lack of Social Contact with Female Peers

Opportunities to interact with females were sparse. Two of the four men lived in group homes housing only males. Planned facility recreational events–such as attending a movie in the community–often did not provide opportunities to meet and interact with individuals from different facility group homes, the facility's campus units, or the facility's apartment program. Consequently, the post-injury activities in which the four men participated not only facilitated isolation but often maintained exclusive contact with other males only. Several of the men reported that their only interaction with women involved the female staff members, whom they perceived to be domineering mother figures, Den Mothers, or prison wardens.

> The female staff here at [name of facility] act like my mother. I don't feel like an adult man. I feel talked down to. Like they're better than me cause they ain't messed up in the head or something. Or cause they work and hold steady jobs. (Sal)

> [Female staff person's name] is like the den mother here. And she thinks we're her prepubescent Boy Scout troop she has to whip into shape. It's a wonder she don't make us raise our hands to take a piss. (Rudy)

Moreover, the men stated that community group home living, rather than facilitating integration, actually inhibited opportunities to meet and interact with females in a naturalistic manner.

> It's stigmatizing being in a community group home. People think I'm disabled. And I can't exactly invite a woman home to dinner or spend the night with a house full of guys with head injuries. (Rudy)

> Even though I'm an independent traveler, a lot of the clients here aren't. And so I can't meet them for dinner at a restaurant because they aren't allowed out. There were a couple of women in the campus units I first met when I came here [to reside at the TBI facility]. But they weren't allowed out without a staff, so I couldn't go out to dinner with them or go to a movie. I'm 44 years old; I don't need no chaperone. (Sal)

Dissatisfaction with Opportunities to Participate in Male Gender Activities

All of the men verbalized dissatisfaction with the opportunities available in the environment to participate in male gender activities. In addition to feeling restricted from sharing activities with females, several of the men expressed that opportunities to engage in satisfying work offering competitive wages were few and far between.

> I'd like to find work that means something to me. Instead of the busywork they give you here [in the facility's sheltered workshop]. It's demeaning to my intelligence to have to put packages of pencils together. (Rudy)

> That's why I volunteer my time, because if I can't get paid decent money for my work then I'd rather donate my time to others. (Sal)

Additionally, all of the men spoke about the lack of opportunity to participate in male gender activities as a result of revoked driving privileges.

> If I could drive again, I could drive to my family's or meet friends. I could drive to go out bowling when I wanted or to a ballgame. And I could get my old job back [as a driver/delivery person]. (Ed)

> Without being able to drive I have no freedom. I'm dependent upon the staff to arrange what they call community outings [Sal gestures quotation symbols with his hands]. I can't socialize with people I'd like to because I can't get over to their residences. (Sal)

Decreased Opportunity to Form an Adult Male Identity

Lacking adequate opportunities in the environment to participate in male gender activities, these men were unable to engage in roles and relationships that could contribute to the formation of a post-injury adult male identity. Opportunities to engage in roles and relationships that could define the men's adult gender identity became particularly important after injury since their adult identity formation was disrupted by the occurrence of TBI. Consequently, several of the men suggested that they did not know themselves as adult men.

> I'm just getting to know me. And I've been living with this head injury for about twenty-some years now. And I still don't really

understand who I am or who I could be. I only have this image of the man I used to be. (Rudy)

I don't really know myself. I haven't had the chance to get to know myself since my injury. My life stopped as how it was. The guy I was, that person is no more. And I'm not sure what's left. (Jay)

ACHIEVEMENT OF RITES OF PASSAGE

Prior to their injuries, most of the four men had achieved several rites of passage into male adulthood. Rites of passage are culture-specific life events that mark the transition from one life stage to another. In western culture, common rites of passage leading to adulthood include obtaining a driver's license, graduating from secondary school or obtaining a degree of higher education, moving out of the parental home, securing full-time employment, establishing an independent residence in the community, dating and establishing initial sexual experiences, marrying, and parenting. All of the men had obtained driver's licenses and completed secondary education; Sal and Jay had earned a year of college credit. Both Sal and Rudy had established successful work histories, and Ed had obtained full-time employment just one year prior to his accident. Sal had realized his goal of home ownership, while Rudy had gained independence by maintaining his own apartment in a large northeastern metropolitan city. Both Sal and Rudy were also independently earning and managing their own finances. With regard to the formation of intimate relationships, Sal had reached his sixth wedding anniversary just prior to his first TBI, and Rudy had engaged in a series of dating relationships.

Loss of an Adult Status

After injury, all of the men had lost the adult status accompanying the rites of passage each achieved pre-injury. Due to the cognitive sequelae of TBI and potential seizure activity, each man lost his driver's license and with that, the adult freedom to travel in society independently. Sal, Rudy, and Ed had lost the ability to engage in their prior work careers. Not only did these men lose professional and trade skills, but they lost their previously established ability to earn a living.

The loss of the ability to work and support oneself financially was perceived by each as a significant loss of adult independence.

> Not being able to work in my trade–work that let me support myself–that's been the biggest blow to myself as a man. Because that means I'm dependent on others. And I don't wanna be dependent on no one. I'm not a child. (Sal)

The inability to maintain an independent residence in the community–and to exert the adult privilege of personal choice within one's home environment–was also perceived as a loss of adult status.

> When I used to live by myself I could do the things that you know, made you feel like an autonomous adult. Like if I wanted to grab a sandwich and a beer and put my feet up and watch a ball game. You can't do that here–it ain't proper [said with sarcasm] to put your feet up on a table. (Rudy)

> I owned my own home. I took care of the property by myself. If something happened I was responsible; I made the decisions. I liked being independent–making decisions for myself instead of living under somebody else's thumb. (Sal)

Inability to Achieve Rites of Passage Post-Injury

In addition to the men's loss of achieved rites of passage into male adulthood, none was able to resume or attain any further rites of passage after injury. It was as if the passage leading to male adulthood in their society had been closed for these men after injury.

> It's like this: This is society [gestures with hands to the environment outside of the group home]. I'm this close to being in society but I'm just looking in. I'm not a member of society. I don't feel like an adult man is supposed to be looked upon in our society. You know, independent, self-supporting, a family man. All the things I'm not. (Rudy)

After injury, Sal and Rudy attempted to resume several rites of passage each had achieved pre-injury but experienced disappointment. Both attempted marriage after injury but divorced shortly after. Rudy attempted to obtain his own apartment in the community but was encouraged by his family to return to a residential rehabilitation program. Sal also had advanced to the apartment program in his present rehabilitation facility but, due to substance abuse and safety issues, was re-assigned to community group home living. The experience of a failed attempt to re-obtain lost rites of passage left these men feeling little hope that they could again enter society as adult men.

> The fact that I lived independently [in the facility's apartment program] and now I had to move back [to a community group home] is disturbing. I feel like I'll never get back the adult independence I had. (Sal)

> I feel like I'm in a hole. And the world is out there and I'm gonna stay in this hole. I try to the best of my capabilities, but it feels like I just can't lift myself outta here. (Rudy)

Feeling Left Behind and Forgotten by Peers and Siblings

A common theme that emerged among all of the men concerned the feeling that their peers and siblings had surpassed them in the achievement of adult male rites of passage. The sentiment, "They have their own lives; I'd only interfere," was expressed frequently and may have reflected feelings of inferiority in comparison to peers' and siblings' attainment of adult roles and relationships.

> The friends I had before my accident got married and had kids; they have their own lives. I don't bother them. . . . I don't visit the friends I made when I lived in the apartments [facility rehabilitation program] either–they look down upon me now cause I was sent back [to a community group home]. (Sal)

> I was always comparing myself to my brother and thinking about his better lifestyle–what he has compared to what I don't have–a family, a business he built himself, a house, the respect of my dad and the community. (Rudy)

> I'm the oldest of five brothers. I should have been married first and had kids. Sometimes I feel jealous. . . . The guys I went to school with also all have wives and kids now. I don't see them; I'd just interfere with their lives. (Ed)

I'd like to be close with my sister–after all, I'm her older brother. But she's above me now–she's getting married. I have some jealousy about her. I understand it–about her better situation. But luckily I'm wise enough to know it's not something I should take out on her. . . . I'd like to see her more but she's doing her own thing. And I respect her need to do that. (Jay)

I think that my friends and family look down upon me. I'm not the productive member of society in their point of view like they probably consider themselves to be. Sometimes I feel like I failed being a man. (Sal)

ADDITIONAL GENDER ROLE STRAIN THEMES

Two further gender role strain themes emerged among the four men: (a) dissatisfaction with their post-injury masculine appearance, and (b) the existence of pre-morbid gender role strain issues. Two of the men–Sal and Rudy–expressed dissatisfaction with their post-injury appearance as adult men. For these men, the ability to appear masculine was an important component of their male gender identity.

I worked construction so I was physically big and strong. I was a bricklayer and I had large muscles. I miss that. Because of the accidents I have chronic pain now. I can't work out physically like I used to cause of the pain–I mean I do minimal weights, but not enough to build any muscle mass worth talk'n about. (Sal)

I used to be much more of an appealing guy. I was more in shape; you know what I mean? I had the physique of an athlete. Now I'm an old man with a limp, a scarred face, a potbelly–who'd want me now? (Rudy)

The ability to appear masculine may have been doubly important for Sal who, as a result of childhood polio, struggled to compensate for an orthopedic deformity involving the vertebral column and lower extremities.

Sal's concern with his post-injury physical appearance emphasizes the importance of considering how the men's experience of post-TBI gender role strain may have been compounded by the existence of pre-morbid gender role strain issues. Several of the other men also reported the possible existence of pre-injury gender role strain issues. Both Ed and Jay did not have the opportunity to form relationships with their biological fathers. Ed's parents failed to disclose the fact that Ed's stepfather was not his biological parent until Ed's adolescence. Despite not having conscious knowledge of his stepfather's true relationship to him, Ed nevertheless reported feeling a distance and estrangement from his stepfather that was not apparent in his stepfather's relationship with Ed's younger brothers. Jay, too, expressed that his relationship with his stepfather while growing up had been conflicted and difficult.

Similarly, while Sal and Rudy reported positive relationships with their fathers, each expressed disappointment regarding distant, strained relationships with their older brothers. Both Sal and Rudy believed that their older brothers were favored offspring whose achievements could not be surpassed. Ed also verbalized resentment regarding his brothers' close relationship with his stepfather. Strained relationships with significant male figures in these men's lives may have compounded post-injury feelings of gender role strain.

The lack of strong male mentors in these men's pre-injury lives continued after they sustained TBI. It is significant that, after injury, none of the men had access to a male mentor having knowledge of the head injury experience who could have served as a guide (e.g., a TBI rehabilitation counselor or an individual with a head injury who successfully rebuilt a satisfactory quality of life). Essentially, the men's experience of head injury must have seemed much like journeying into the unknown. They were traveling a path that other men with head injury had traversed, but without having access to those individuals' knowledge and insight.

Chapter 4

The Intervention Process:
A Description of the Treatment Methods
Used to Alleviate Gender Role Strain

The four men received occupational therapy for four months to help
them rebuild the desired male gender roles that they had lost–or never
attained–as a result of their TBI. The occupational therapy intervention process was based on a specific set of guidelines for practice:
"Enhancing Gender Role Satisfaction in Adult Males with Traumatic
Brain Injury" (Gutman, 1997). This set of guidelines is intended to be
used with men who sustained TBI at 18-30 years of age and who are
currently at least two years post-injury. The two-year anniversary date
seems to be a time when individuals begin to understand how their
lives have changed as a result of TBI. It is a time when individuals are
more willing to relinquish some of the denial that commonly accom-
panies a traumatic injury and impedes the rehabilitation process. Denial is often used initially to lessen the psychological impact of having
sustained a severe injury that alters the course of one's life. In this
way, denial is useful, as it enables individuals to maintain hope and to
remain motivated to participate in therapy. However, when denial is
used excessively–that is, when individuals deny that they have any
deficits as a result of injury–denial becomes problematic and prevents
the individual from making gains in the rehabilitation process.

By two years post-TBI, much of the physical recovery stage is

[Haworth co-indexing entry note]: "The Intervention Process: A Description of the Treatment Methods
Used to Alleviate Gender Role Strain." Gutman, Sharon A. Co-published simultaneously in *Occupational
Therapy in Mental Health* (The Haworth Press, Inc.) Vol. 15, No. 3/4, 2000, pp. 49-66; and: *Brain Injury
and Gender Role Strain: Rebuilding Adult Lifestyles After Injury* (Sharon A. Gutman) The Haworth Press,
Inc., 2000, pp. 49-66. Single or multiple copies of this article are available for a fee from The Haworth
Document Delivery Service [1-800-342-9678, 9:00 a.m. - 5:00 p.m. (EST). E-mail address: getinfo@haworth
pressinc.com].

49

complete. While individuals can continue to progress in physical skills throughout the remainder of their lives, physical recovery commonly slows after the two-year mark. However, psychosocial sequelae become readily apparent when physical recovery begins to slow. Because the physical deficits of brain injury are visible, patients and healthcare professionals tend to focus on physical deficits during the initial years of rehabilitation. It is only when the physical recovery process begins to lessen in intensity that individuals tend to become more aware of the psychosocial and emotional problems associated with TBI. At the two-year point, males with TBI tend to become more readily aware of the adult male roles they have lost–or have been unable to attain–as a result of TBI. Feelings of gender role strain become apparent at two years post-TBI (Fleming & Strong, 1999).

THE INTERVENTION SETTING

The occupational therapy intervention that the four men received can be administered in both group and one-to-one sessions. The intervention appears to be administered best in a TBI rehabilitation facility (e.g., a residential or day program) in which individuals have ready access to a community of staff and fellow clients with whom to rebuild networks of gender social roles and activities. The four men described in this book lived in a residential rehabilitation facility for adults with TBI. The facility was located in a suburb of a large northeastern metropolitan city and was easily accessible to shopping, restaurants, and recreation (e.g., movie theaters, parks, malls). Because individuals in the post-acute stages of TBI commonly experience a variety of physical, cognitive, and psychosocial sequelae and often possess vastly different functional levels, the facility was designed to accommodate varying client needs through multiple types of residences:

A. Clients who required moderate to maximum assistance for the performance of basic daily living skills (e.g., bathing, dressing, eating, toileting) resided in one of three main facility *campus units that provided 24 hour staff supervision.* Each campus unit resembled a ranch house with a large kitchen, laundry, dining room, recreation room, and 10 shared dormitory rooms (for 2 clients) with their own bathroom. The front and back entrances of the building opened onto garden patios. Each building housed approximately 16 clients. The three ranch house residences shared a 10 acre campus with a vocational workshop, administration building, and a therapy building. The administration and therapy buildings were part of a renovated 19th century manor house and stable. The campus resembled an old-world European village in which everyone knew each other and the days maintained their own rhythm, separate from the outside world beyond the stone pillars that framed the campus entrance.

B. Four *community group homes* were located near the main facility campus but were ensconced within the residential community neighborhoods that sat adjacent to the main campus. Each community group home housed five to six individuals who required only distant staff supervision for self-care activities, but close staff supervision for more complex daily living skills (e.g., meal preparation, banking and money management, and the use of public transportation). Each client had his own bedroom in the house and was responsible for the upkeep of his personal room, laundry, and a rotating weekly chore (e.g., vacuuming the family room, cleaning the bathroom, loading the dishwasher). Meals were provided by the facility and clients typically shared dinner at a common time, seated together at a large family dining room table stationed in each of the four homes. Often staff members prepared dinners–assisted by one or more clients–and joined the clients in the sharing of the meal. Some evenings were spent together watching rented videos in the house's family room. Individuals who resided in the community group homes often worked in the facility's vocational workshop (alongside some of the clients who resided in the campus units) or were able–through vocational training–to assume paid employment or a volunteer position in the community.

C. The facility additionally housed approximately 15 individuals in *dual occupancy community apartments*. Like the community group homes, these apartments were also located in a residential neighborhood near the main campus, but farther away than the group home locations. Individuals who were able to live in the shared apartments commonly required only 12 hours of distant supervision for higher level daily living skills and could often use public transportation independently. Most of the apartment program residents were employed in the community and could obtain their own groceries and prepare meals independently.

The four men in this book resided in the community group homes (each in a separate residence), but did not commonly interact with one another. Each man transitioned through a progression of residences beginning with an initial admission to the campus units. As they progressed in rehabilitation and relearned daily living skills, each had been transferred to community group living. Only Sal had advanced in rehabilitation far enough to achieve shared community apartment living, but had been transferred back to the group homes as a result of risk-taking behaviors in a less supervised environment. In the culture of the TBI facility, clients who resided in the apartments held the highest status and were admired, or envied, by clients living in the group homes–much like the established pecking order amongst college seniors living in frat houses and freshman relegated to dormitories. Conversely, clients who resided in the community group homes were the envy of those living in the campus units, waiting for the chance to move from the ranch-like institution to a nondescript group home in a residential neighborhood.

INDICATIONS/CONTRAINDICATIONS

The intervention that the four men received is indicated for individuals who exhibit no more than minimal to moderate confusion, display a moderate capacity for the integration of new learning, and require no greater than minimal to moderate assistance for most activities of daily living. The use of this intervention is contraindicated with individuals who exhibit severe cognitive deficits and are unable to demonstrate the integration of new learning.

DESCRIPTION OF THE INTERVENTION

A set of guidelines for practice is a collection of treatment principles designed to ameliorate a specific clinical condition. In other words, a set of guidelines for practice describes an intervention process. Sets of guidelines for clinical practice provide direction for problem identification (or assessment) and remediation (or treatment). The instructions for problem identification and remediation are derived from both (a) theoretical information accepted by the scientific community and (b) clinical observation of patient populations having specific medical/psychosocial conditions.

THEORETICAL BASE OF THE INTERVENTION

The theoretical base of a set of guidelines for practice provides empirical support for problem identification and resolution of a specific clinical problem. A theoretical base is derived from theory or empirical data that describe the characteristics of the clinical problem specified. The theoretical information that provides support for the set of guidelines described in this book was drawn from (a) gender role theory, (b) social role acquisition theory, and (c) social learning theory. Information from these theories was used to construct the procedures for both problem identification and remediation of post-TBI gender role strain.

Gender is an identification of oneself and others as male or female. Humans express their gender identity through social roles and activities that are perceived to possess masculine and/or feminine qualities. The perception of social roles and activities as having masculine and/or feminine qualities is culturally determined. While gender identity is the internal perception of oneself as a male or female, gender roles provide the social relationships and activities through which an individual's gender identity can be expressed (Money, 1994).

Gender identity and role development begin at birth and continue throughout maturation. As children begin to internalize cultural definitions of gender, they learn to use gender as a lens through which all social information is interpreted. In western society, the family of origin, childhood peer groups, school systems, and the media participate in the socialization of children into male and female gender roles (Bem, 1993).

By early adulthood, most individuals have developed consistent and stable gender identities. However, when individuals transition from one life stage to another, they also change the social roles and activities that support their gender roles as a male or female. For example, heterosexual males who transition from childhood to adolescence often change their social roles and activities from the exclusive participation in same sex-oriented activities (e.g., participating in all male sports teams) to the inclusion of opposite sex-oriented activities (such as dating). Changes in the activities and social roles that support one's gender role must be developmentally appropriate to the new life stage. However, when males sustain TBI between the ages of 18-30, the transition from adolescence to adulthood is disrupted. Males who sustain TBI between the years of 18-30 can find that the acquisition of adult male gender roles can be permanently disrupted. It is this inability to assume the desired gender roles of male adulthood after the occurrence of a TBI that appears to lead to male gender role strain.

Gender role strain occurs when an individual experiences difficulty in three primary areas of human experience: (a) the participation in gender social roles, (b) the participation in gender activities, and (c) the achievement of gender rites of passage. Common gender social roles of male adulthood in western society include familial roles (e.g., husband, father, son, brother) and extended-family roles, courtship or dating roles, community member roles (e.g., worker, volunteer, organization member), mentor-protégé roles, and friend roles. Extended-family roles are non-biological/non-legal relationships between individuals that mirror the functions of biological/legal family relationships when familial relationships are inaccessible to the individual.

The intervention was designed to assist males with TBI to engage in the above male gender social roles. For example, in the intervention, mentor-protégé roles are developed within relationships between a man with TBI and a male clinical professional who is willing to make a commitment to guide the psychosocial development of the client in a caring, one-to-one relationship for a period of the client's participation in rehabilitation. Professional-client, mentor-protégé relationships are intended to mirror the teacher/student or coach/athlete relationships commonly found between middle-aged and young adult men. Mentors can also be other men with TBI who have successfully rebuilt their post-injury lives and are willing to mentor other men with TBI who could benefit from the insight and guidance offered by individuals who have first hand knowledge of the TBI experience.

The set of guidelines was also designed to assist males with TBI to achieve the rites of passage marking the transition from male adolescence to adulthood. The achievement of adult male rites of passage is dependent upon an individual's ability to first assume specific male gender roles and activities.

Rites of passage are culturally specific and publicly acknowledged events that mark the transition from one life stage to another (Davies, 1994; Diasio-Serrett, Schallert, & Shively, 1994). The transition from male adolescence to adulthood in western society is often marked by such socially acknowledged rites of passage as obtaining a driver's license, engaging in initial sexual experiences, graduating from secondary or higher education, leaving the parental home, securing employment, getting married, and becoming a father. These rites of passage often become inaccessible to individuals whose TBI occurred during the developmental transition from adolescence to adulthood. In western society, as in most cultures, male adulthood is a status to be achieved. The achievement of male adulthood is publicly marked by the above noted rites of passage. When these rites of passage cannot be achieved after injury, males with TBI commonly report a sense of lost male adulthood.

Rites of passage are social events that depend upon the community's public acknowledgement of an individual's newly achieved social status (Grimes, 1995). It is the public acknowledgement of a newly acquired social status that lends the achieved status its meaning. Ceremonial events involved in the marking of rites of passage–in all human cultures–are intended to invite the individual to further participate in the community as an adult member. Such traditional rites of passage may require modification in order to be achieved by an individual with TBI. When the achievement of traditional rites of passage is not possible, however, individuals are encouraged to adopt nontraditional rites of passage that may also provide meaning and a sense of male adulthood.

Because desired adult male gender roles and activities must be assumed before one can transition through a specific adult rite of passage, most of the four men in this book worked on regaining the skills to rebuild important male gender social roles and activities. The achievement of specific adult male rites of passage began to occur near the end of the four-month intervention and continued after the formal intervention period had been completed.

BEHAVIORS INDICATIVE OF DYSFUNCTION

Listed below is a behavioral guide to the identification of gender role strain. The presence of the following behaviors is used to determine the existence and severity of gender role strain. You may recognize these behaviors in yourself if you are a man with TBI, in your loved one if you are a family member of a man with TBI, or in your clients if you are a health care professional.

Deficits in the Ability to Assume Male Gender **Social Roles**

A. *The individual is unable to participate in more than one half of the activities that supported his male gender role prior to injury.*

Pre-injury adult roles such as worker/student, sports participant, and independent home maintainer have been lost and have become difficult to rebuild after injury due to the individual's physical, cognitive, and psychosocial sequelae.

B. *The individual is unable to rebuild the adult male gender social roles that supported his pre-injury relationships.* The individual's loss of such roles as husband/boyfriend, father, brother, son, and uncle has disrupted his ability to maintain meaningful relationships formed prior to his injury. Consequently, the individual reports that the opportunities in his environment and family system to participate in adult male roles have been closed off to him.

C. *The individual becomes isolated and lacks opportunities to socialize with others.* Because the individual has lost the pre-injury social roles that once supported meaningful relationships with others, the individual now finds that he is unable to rebuild pre-injury relationships and cannot form and sustain new relationships after injury. Consequently, the individual reports that he feels abandoned by close friends and family members.

D. *The individual participates in gender social roles characteristic of adolescence or an earlier developmental period.* Either (a) the individual has been unable to adopt adult male gender roles after an injury that occurred during the transition from adolescence to adulthood or (b) if the individual had been able to adopt several adult male gender roles pre-injury, he has not been able to maintain them post-injury. The individual reports feeling more like an adolescent than an adult man, or he may perceive that others consider him to be an adolescent rather than an adult.

Deficits in the Ability to Assume Adult Male Gender **Activities**

A. *The individual has lost more than one half of the adult male gender social roles that he established prior to his injury.* Pre-injury activities such as dating (sexual intimacy), sports participation, and mechanically oriented work (the repair of cars, home renovation)–which supported the individual's role as an adult man–have been lost as a result of injury. The inability to participate in these activities may be due to (a) the physical, cognitive, and/or psychosocial sequelae * of TBI, and/or (b) a lack of opportunity in the environment to participate in adult male activities.

B. *After injury, the individual has been unable to adopt new activities that could support his role as an adult man.* The individual's inability to adopt new activities after injury may be due to a lack of exposure to alternative post-injury activities that could replace lost pre-injury activities. The individual may also believe that pre-injury activities alone can provide a sense of male adulthood.

C. *The individual continues to participate in activities that are characteristic of adolescence or an earlier developmental period.* The inability to adopt the activities of male adulthood is often due to a brain injury that occurred during the individual's transition from adolescence to adulthood. Essentially, the individual appears to be stuck in adolescence and the activities and roles that are characteristic of adolescence.

D. *The individual may also participate in activities that facilitate exclusive contact with others outside of the individual's own developmental life-stage.* In other words, although the individual is the chronological age of an adult man, his injury occurred during adolescence. Consequently, because he has been unable to transition from adolescence to adulthood he feels most comfortable interacting with adolescents and participating in adolescent activities.

E. *The individual participates in activities that facilitate social isolation or exclusive contact with a single gender group.* For example, the individual may engage in isolative activities such as watching television or listening to music alone in his room. The individual may also live in an all-male community group home that does not provide sufficient opportunity to interact with female peers.

F. *The individual does not engage in a sufficient amount of daily activities that are able to fill his day.* Consequently, the individual often spends 3-5 hours of daytime hours without any activity (e.g., sleeping, sitting silently in a chair).

Deficits in the Ability to Achieve Adult Male **Rites of Passage**

A. *The individual who was able to achieve several adult male rites of passage prior to injury (e.g., obtaining a driver's license, living independently in the community, obtaining full-time employment, dating and engaging in sexual relationships) is unable to maintain the adult status that had originally accompanied these rites of passage.* Rites of passage mark the transition from one life stage to another. The individual who achieved several adult rites of passage prior to his injury originally gained the status of an adult man. After injury, the status of adulthood was stripped from him because of his inability to resume his former adult roles and relationships, and his dependency on others. The individual may now be a 40 year old man who is treated by others like an adolescent. When staff and family members treat adult men like adolescents, they inadvertently participate in the stripping of his adult status.

B. *The individual is unable to continue his transition from adolescence to adulthood by achieving further common adult rites of passage after injury.* Often individuals with TBI who have achieved several rites of passage prior to injury find that they are unable to further achieve specific rites of passage including marriage/forming a committed relationship, parenting, career expansion, independent community living, and mentoring of a younger protégé.

DIRECTIONS TO PROMOTE POSITIVE CHANGE

The directions to promote positive change describe the treatment steps that are carried out in the intervention process. The set of guidelines consists of three tiers of directions: (a) the first tier addresses the skills necessary for men with TBI to rebuild desired gender **social roles,** (b) the second tier addresses the skills necessary to resume desired gender **activities,** and (c) the third tier helps men achieve desired **rites of passage** into adulthood.

These tiers are arranged in a developmental order in accordance with a progressive treatment sequence. Treatment begins by determining which gender social roles are desired by the individual and by then encouraging him to choose specific activities that could support the acquisition of the identified gender roles. Because the ability to achieve rites of passage is dependent upon the assumption of self-identified roles and activities, the tier addressing rites of passage should be addressed last.

Tier 1:   Identify male gender **social roles** that the individual wishes to rebuild (or build anew).

Tier 2:   Identify the **activities** that could support desired social roles.

Tier 3:   Identify the adult **rites of passage** that the individual wishes to achieve.

Tier 1: Directions to Promote the Rebuilding of Desired Adult Male **Social Roles**

A. *Help the individual to develop ways to actively engage more fully in his pre-injury established familial roles.* For example, an individual who lives apart from his family in a residential treatment program may engage in his role as a brother through the medium of telephone calls, e-mail, letter writing, and using public transportation to visit family members. The individual may need to relearn specific social skills to interact with loved ones. For example, a father with TBI who has low frustration tolerance and is bothered by noise secondary to TBI, will benefit from an opportunity to relearn the social and play skills necessary to interact with his children.

B. *Help the individual to create extended-family relationships with other individuals if the biological/legal family relationships are not existent or accessible.* Brain injury can tear families apart. Often individuals with TBI report estrangement from loved ones after their accidents. Such individuals will benefit greatly from the formation of extended-family relationships with other clients in the rehabilitation center, support group, or day program. Extended-family relationships are non-biological/non-legal relationships that offer a sense of affinity for individuals who feel estranged from biological/legal family members.

C. *Help the individual to develop one-to-one mentor-protégé relationships with a same-gender rehabilitation professional who can offer appropriate guidance and insight into the brain injury experience.* An individual who has a brain injury and has successfully rebuilt his life after injury can also act as a mentor who can provide insight from first hand knowledge of what it's like to live with a brain injury. The mentor-protégé relationship is intended to mirror coach/athlete or teacher/student relationships in which an experienced male mentor provides emotional support, advice derived from experience, and friendship to a less experienced male who is in an earlier stage of TBI rehabilitation.

D. *Help the individual to develop same-gender and cross-gender friendships.* One of the most detrimental affects of TBI is the social isolation that commonly occurs after injury. It is important to help men with TBI to develop a network of friends that includes both men and women. Men with TBI often report that their male buddy friendships are lost after injury. Consequently, men with TBI not only lose male friends with whom to participate in male gender activities (e.g., sports events) but they also lose male friends with whom they can discuss personal concerns and problems. It is also critical to help men with TBI to develop friendships with females as well–as males often report that their opportunity to interact with females is significantly reduced after injury. Males with TBI need female peers with whom to engage in friendships. Such friendships provide the opportunity for the demonstration of compassion and caring–feelings that may not as easily emerge within male-male friendships.

E. *Help the individual to facilitate dating relationships.* The dating/courtship role is an important role for individuals who sustained their TBI between 18-30 years old–particularly if the occurrence of the TBI facilitated the end of a committed relationship or marriage. Many heterosexual men whose TBI occurred between 18-30 years old report that they have been unable to establish intimate relationships with women after their injury. Opportunities to meet women who are suitable dating partners are limited. Often men with TBI who live in residential programs reside in all-male group homes. Many such men report that their only interactions with women are with the female staff members and therapists. It will likely be important to help men with TBI to relearn the appropriate social interaction skills necessary for dating relationships. The facilitation of dating relationships, however, must be implemented in a supportive environment. Residential assisted living arrangements should provide privacy, transportation to recreation (movies, restaurants), safe sex education, and ongoing counseling to deal with the everyday strains of intimate relationships (particularly ones compounded by brain injury).

F. *Help the individual to regain the community member role.* Belonging to a community in which one can find purpose, meaning, friendship, and an adult status is critically important for the individual who feels that his TBI has closed the doors to a position in the larger community outside of the treatment center. Before their injury, many men reported that they found a sense of meaning and belonging through such communities as school/work, religious organizations, developmental and/or charitable groups (e.g., Scouts, Masons), and volunteer groups (e.g., Town Watch, Habitat For Humanity). Often such community member roles–particularly the worker/student role–are closed off for individuals with TBI due to their physical, cognitive, and psychosocial sequelae. Men with TBI who cannot regain the community member role report that they feel that their society has rejected them. It is important for these men to regain community member roles in order to facilitate a sense of belonging, an adult status, and a feeling that their contributions are valued by others. Community member role opportunities for men with TBI can include becoming a public advocate for safe driving (e.g., speaking to students in the school system), volunteer positions in nursing homes or public libraries, and participating in community college courses. The opportunity to contribute to the larger society through a volunteer position becomes crucially important for men with TBI, as employment that is both personally satisfying and well paying is often difficult to obtain after injury.

Tier 2: Directions to Promote the Participation in Desired **Adult Male Activities**

A. *Adult activities that the individual used to support his male gender role before his injury should be adapted so that he can participate in desired activities despite deficits secondary to TBI.* For example, specific sports can be modified to allow individuals with disabilities to participate–e.g., wheelchair basketball; musical performance can be modified for individuals with poor fine motor coordination by using electronic equipment.

B. *Individuals should also be provided with opportunities to observe and participate in novel adult activities never before engaged in prior to injury.* Such exposure to new activities can increase the individual's awareness of post-injury activities that could replace lost pre-injury activities. This is particularly important for the man who believes that the resumption of his former, pre-injury activities is the only way to regain a sense of male adulthood. Such an individual might miss important opportunities to participate in new activities that could provide a sense of male adulthood.

C. *It is also important to help the individual to identify adult activities that could socially connect him to others* (particularly others belonging to the same developmental age group). Because social isolation is the most frequently reported psychosocial problem after brain injury, activities that promote social interaction with similar others is necessary for a successful TBI rehabilitation. TBI social support groups that meet for dinner or day trips and sporting events for individuals with TBI are two examples of popular activities that can both facilitate a sense of male adulthood and socially connect the individual to others (both men and women).

Tier 3:	Directions to Promote the Achievement of **Rites of Passage** That Mark the Transition into Male Adulthood

First, the individual must identify desired rites of passage into male adulthood. It will be likely that these will fall into two categories–those that are realistic and easily achievable, and those that may not be (for example, re-obtaining one's driver's license when one requires seizure medication and possesses visual-perceptual deficits). When desired rites of passage cannot be obtained, it becomes necessary to help the individual to create nontraditional rites of passage that may also be personally meaningful.

A. *It becomes important to help the individual to adapt traditional rites of passage to make their achievement more feasible.* For example, a traditional rite of passage into male adulthood is marrying and assuming the role of a husband. The rite of marriage may be adapted by allowing unmarried adults who are their own legal guardians to live together in a monogamous, committed relationship within the supportive environment of a residential TBI program. The rite of obtaining a driver's license may be adapted by teaching the individual to use public transportation independently.

B. *Additionally, nontraditional rites of passage should be created when the traditional ones cannot be adapted.* For example, a traditional rite of adulthood is the attainment of independent living in the community. One adaptation of independent community living for individuals who require supervised assisted living arrangements is the attainment of a private room in a community group home residence after one has shared personal space with a roommate on a facility ward housing 15 other individuals.

C. *Because rites of passage gain their status from public acknowledgement, it is important to celebrate (or in some way publicly acknowledge) an individual's attainment of a desired rite of passage into adulthood.* When an individual achieves an adapted and/or nontraditional rite of passage into adulthood, the community (e.g., the TBI program, the immediate family) should acknowledge the individual's newly gained adult status with (a) greater adult privileges, (b) official chart documentation, and/or (c) a celebration/ceremony. Such acknowledgement signifies to the individual that his community recognizes his adult status.

General Directions to Facilitate Tier 1, 2, and 3

Additionally, sets of guidelines for practice contain **general directions** that are intended to facilitate each identified tier of skills.

A. *The individual should be provided with the opportunity to observe others (who share the same approximate age and role expectations) as they participate in desired social roles and activities in both simulated (e.g., TV, film) and natural environments (e.g., the community mall, restaurants).* Observing similar others encourages the individual to believe that if others can learn specific skills, he can as well.

B. *The individual should be offered the opportunity to role-play the use of specific desired skills with the therapist* (e.g., how to act on a date; how to act as an uncle to one's toddler nephew). Role-playing allows the individual to practice desired skills with a professional in a safe non-threatening environment (e.g., the treatment center).

C. *The individual should also be encouraged to practice specific desired skills in both simulated and natural settings.* Practice should begin in simulated settings to decrease the anxiety that may be produced by having to learn an unfamiliar skill. When skills are mastered in simulated settings, therapy should then move toward the practice of skills in natural settings that the individual is likely to encounter.

D. *It is necessary for the individual to receive ongoing feedback from the therapist in order to refine desired skills overtime.*

E. *It is also necessary to provide sufficient opportunity for the individual to repeatedly practice desired skills until learned.*

METHODS OF DATA COLLECTION
REGARDING INTERVENTION OUTCOMES

In order to assess the effectiveness of the intervention with each of the four men, interviews regarding the severity of each man's gender role strain were conducted (a) prior to the four-month intervention, (b) once weekly during the intervention period, and (c) two weeks after the end of the intervention. Interviews were conducted by occupational therapy students who were trained in interview methods.

The pre-intervention questions address the severity of each man's gender role strain. These initial questions provided a baseline against which change in gender role strain could be compared after the intervention was completed. The concurrent-intervention questions were asked on a weekly basis during the four-month intervention period. The post-intervention questions were asked to determine whether changes in each man's gender role strain/satisfaction occurred after his participation in the intervention.

Pre-Intervention Interview Questions

1. What were your expectations for your adult life prior to your injury (with regard to work, family, hobbies, residential conditions, dating/marriage, etc.)?
2. Presently, have you met these expectations? Have you been able to create a post-injury lifestyle that is personally satisfactory? Why/why not?
3. Have your expectations changed since injury? In what ways?
4. Presently, what are your most important roles (e.g., worker, husband/boyfriend, friend, community volunteer, sports enthusiast, etc.)?
5. What roles did you participate in prior to your injury (i.e., family, friend, work, dating/courtship, and community member roles)? Which of these roles supported your identity as an adult man?
6. Do you still participate in these roles? How do you feel about having lost some of these roles?
7. What activities did you participate in prior to your injury? Which of these activities supported your identity as an adult man? Have you lost any of these activities? How does the loss of these activities make you feel?
8. What new roles and activities did you begin to participate in after your injury? Do these activities enable you to think of yourself as an adult man? Describe a typical day for you.
9. Who are your closest friends and family members? What types of activities do you share with these people?
10. Has your relationship with your family, spouse/girlfriend, children, friends, etc., changed after your injury? In what ways? How have these changes affected you?
11. Are there activities that you would like to participate in, but are presently unable to?

12. Do you feel that there is adequate opportunity in your environment to participate in all of the roles and activities that you would like to?
13. Do you feel that that there is adequate opportunity to participate in your community as an adult man? Do you feel that others treat you like an adult?
14. How independent do you feel in your present living arrangements?
15. Do you feel that you are able to make your own choices and decisions? Why/why not?
16. Do you feel in control of your life?
17. Do you interact with siblings and pre-injury friends since your injury? Is there a change in your post-injury relationships with old friends and siblings? Can you describe these changes and what they mean to you?

Concurrent-Intervention Interview Questions

1. Which gender roles did you participate in during the previous week?
2. How often during the week did you participate in each of these roles?
3. What activities were associated with each role?
4. Which family members did you interact with this week?
5. Which community member roles did you participate in?
6. Which friends did you get a chance to see?
7. How personally satisfying was each of these roles?
8. Was there enough time to spend with the people you care about?
9. Which roles enable you to feel like an adult man?
10. Which roles make you feel the most comfortable? Which roles are experienced with discomfort?
11. Which roles would you like to participate in more often/less often?
12. Are there any other roles–that you didn't mention–that would enable you to feel more like an adult man?

Post-Intervention Interview Questions

1. Which roles do you have in your present life?
2. How satisfying and personally meaningful are these roles?

3. Do these roles enable you to feel like an adult man?
4. Do you feel that others view you as an adult man?
5. Have you achieved any personal goals recently? Can you describe them? How did it feel to achieve these goals?
6. Do you feel like a part of your community/society? In what ways?
7. Do you feel that you can contribute to others? Do you feel that others value your contributions?
8. What expectations do you have for yourself that you'd still like to fulfill?
9. Do you feel a sense of personal control in your life? Are you able to make your own choices and decisions?
10. Who do you feel most comfortable with and why?
11. Do you feel that others accept you for who you are?
12. How competent do you feel in your daily life activities (which specific activities)?

Chapter 5

Each Man's Intervention Story:
Rebuilding a Satisfying Adult Life
After TBI

The intervention for each of the four men is described using a case study format. As an occupational therapist, I provided much of the treatment intervention with the assistance of a rehabilitation counselor (who was employed at the TBI facility) and several other health care professionals who were committed to helping these men enhance their post-injury lives. We primarily addressed Tier 1 and 2 of the intervention guidelines: that is, helping the men (a) to rebuild desired adult male gender roles (Tier 1) and (b) to resume desired adult male activities (Tier 2). The rebuilding of roles and activities is necessary before one can achieve desired rites of passage (which is addressed by Tier 3 of the intervention). However, some of the men did begin to achieve desired adult rites of passage near the completion of the four-month intervention. The two headings–Adult Male Gender Roles (Tier 1) and Adult Male Activities (Tier 2)–are used to organize the following description of each man's intervention process.

JAY: THE CREATIVE WRITER.
THE ASSUMPTION OF ADULT MALE
GENDER ROLES (TIER 1)

At the time that Jay sustained his injury, he was a college sophomore who had not as yet assumed roles of male adulthood. Although

[Haworth co-indexing entry note]: "Each Man's Intervention Story: Rebuilding a Satisfying Adult Life After TBI." Gutman, Sharon A. Co-published simultaneously in *Occupational Therapy in Mental Health* (The Haworth Press, Inc.) Vol. 15, No. 3/4, 2000, pp. 67-110; and: *Brain Injury and Gender Role Strain: Rebuilding Adult Lifestyles After Injury* (Sharon A. Gutman) The Haworth Press, Inc., 2000, pp. 67-110. Single or multiple copies of this article are available for a fee from The Haworth Document Delivery Service [1-800-342-9678, 9:00 a.m. - 5:00 p.m. (EST). E-mail address: getinfo@haworthpressinc.com].

67

as a child and adolescent, Jay struggled with obsessive compulsive disorder (OCD) and attention deficit hyperactivity disorder (ADHD), in college he had begun to discover successful strategies to sublimate his high energy level and distractible attention span through creative pursuits. His considerable intellectual skills and writing abilities were well suited to his chosen college major of journalism and communications. In his first year of college, Jay began to value his creative gifts and recognized that he could both connect to others and contribute to the larger community through his writing–two important social tasks he found to be difficult due to his distractibility, hyperactivity, and rigid requirements for objects in his environment.

As a white, middle-class, heterosexual male, Jay expected to obtain a college degree and embark upon a career that would afford him the opportunity to participate in the larger society as an independent, self-supporting adult man. The occurrence of his TBI altered his ability to assume the kind of work role that Jay envisioned for himself pre-injury. Because members of Jay's treatment team–like many TBI rehabilitation professionals–believed that resumption of the work role was a highly valuable component of all TBI rehabilitation, Jay was placed in the facility's sheltered workshop to perform piecework 3-5 hours per day, Monday through Friday. While Jay's head injury compounded his distractibility and caused him to experience severe short-term memory deficits, it did not alter his level of intelligence; Jay found his engagement in piecework to be demeaning and intellectually unstimulating. At the time of the intervention, Jay had lost hope that he could participate in an adult work role that was both personally meaningful and able to provide expression of his creative talents.

Jay had not engaged in writing since his accident. Like many males with ADHD, Jay was left hand dominant–a neurologic phenomenon that has been shown to possess statistical significance (Miller, 1990). Left hand dominance–as well as all left sided movement of the body–is caused by dominance of the right neural hemisphere. Some theorists speculate that learning disabilities result from a developmental lag occurring in the left neural hemisphere. The left neural hemisphere is believed to be responsible for concrete functions including math and the literal interpretation of language (as required in reading). Conversely, the right neural hemisphere–which mediates abstract spatial skills and creative abilities–can often develop in a highly sophisticated manner. Consequently, the concomitant advanced development

of the right neural hemisphere and underdevelopment of the left hemisphere is believed to be a predisposing factor of learning disability
(Geschwind & Galaburda, 1987). Interestingly, because right hemi-
spheral development occurs more quickly and fully than left, individuals with learning disabilities are also likely to be left hand dominant.

After injury, Jay–who had been left hand dominant pre-injury–was
forced to switch hand dominance as a result of left upper extremity
spasticity (abnormally increased muscle tone) secondary to neurologic
injury. Unfortunately, Jay experienced writing with his right hand to
be cumbersome and found that he could not record his thoughts quickly enough before his short-term memory deficits interfered with recall.

It was curious that Jay had not been exposed to the use of computers–
other than computer games and rote activities–during his rehabilitation. Computer word processing programs appeared to be a logical
tool to compensate for Jay's upper extremity fine motor difficulties. It
is possible that Jay's therapists believed that he no longer possessed
the language ability to write after injury. It is also likely that no one
questioned Jay concerning his personal goals for the assumption of
particular adult male roles. Therapists on Jay's treatment team may not
have considered that writing was a part of Jay's identity as an adult
worker, since it was unlikely that he would use his post-injury writing
to procure an income.

Jay, however, viewed the opportunity to begin writing again as a
chance to assume a meaningful work role–regardless of whether he
used his writing to earn money. Using an adapted computer system
(described below) and minimal assistance from his therapist, Jay produced short stories and narratives in which he described his experience
of head injury, wrote a letter to the National Brain Injury Association
requesting resource information, and composed poetry as gifts for family members. One of Jay's self-identified milestones occurred when he
wrote and submitted a piece of poetry to a magazine for individuals
sharing the experience of chronic disability (see Figure 5.1). In this
poem, Jay invited others to understand how his life had been altered by
TBI, and in doing so, extended part of himself to a larger community of
others who could benefit from his insight and observations.

> I feel like an adult again, using the computer to express myself. I
> didn't think I'd write again after my accident. It feels really good

to act in an adult way–to create something that other people seem to respect and value me for.

Jay's rehabilitation treatment team members were so impressed with Jay's computer usage and writing pursuits that they featured him in a facility-sponsored newsletter. Additionally, Jay received similar praise when he read aloud a marriage prayer he had written for his sister's upcoming wedding (see Figure 5.2). Jay was not only beginning to re-create his role as a writer, he was attempting to use his writing to re-enter his role within his family system.

As mentioned, Jay reported feeling alienated from his family members before and after ʹinjury. He expressed both jealousy regarding his sister's imminent marriage and anxiety that he would not be included in the wedding plans–as were other members of the immediate family. When Jay wrote the wedding prayer for his sister, he did so with the hope of resolving some of his own jealousy by contributing a part of himself to the couple's union. As a brother, Jay was essentially asking permission to enter and become a member of the couple's new family system. Jay's sister, however, was so moved by his writing that she requested Jay to read it aloud as part of the actual ceremony. In this way, Jay was able to use his writing to re-establish his role as a brother.

> I really wanted to be part of the wedding–I mean as [my sister's] brother. And do the brotherly things you do at weddings. And writing the marriage prayer was, I guess you could say it was a creative solution.

Jay also created additional solutions to engage more actively in his role as a brother. Through an adapted e-mail program (described below), Jay began to correspond regularly with his sister and two cousins living on the West Coast. Jay's ability to use his e-mail program independently meant that he could establish contact with chosen family members when he desired–rather than waiting for contact to be externally initiated. This volitional control enabled Jay to moderate his interaction with family members in accordance with his own comfort level. Moreover, acting upon his volition further meant that Jay could actually observe his control over the re-entry into his family system.

> E-mail is better than the phone because, well, number one, I can't afford that many long distance calls. And [sister's name] lives in

California anyway so she may not be awake when I want to call. But with e-mail I can make instant contact whenever I want. And it's contact that I initiated, so it's not like I'm sitting around waiting and hoping for [my family members] to get in contact with me.

The other thing with e-mail is that it allows me time to think. I say wiser things on e-mail than just by talking face-to-face sometimes. I mean, it [e-mail] allows me to think about what I'd like to say–to compose my thoughts more.

FIGURE 5.1. Jay's Poetry Describing His Experience of Head Injury

Published Poem

The farthest from this earth that I've gone has been the coma,
And then I awoke and consciousness emerged.
It was like being placed in a country for which I had neither the language nor the passport,
And I had lost my I.D. as well.
A part of me died during the car crash.
It's harder now to escape my enemies–being stagnant and accepting mediocrity in myself.
I'm learning about myself now, which is similar to discovering uncharted territory within my soul.
My positive thinking has given me fuel for this challenging and uplifiing journey.
I feel excited and intrigued by all of the imagined and not yet imagined possible opportunities just around the bend.

Reprinted with permission.

FIGURE 5.2. Jay's Wedding Poem to His Sister and Brother-in-Law Illustrating His Ability to Use His Writing to Become a Part of the Wedding

Dear Andrew and Sarah,
I hope that your marriage allows the uniqueness and individuality of each of you to come forth.
And that by allowing each other to be an individual, your marriage will grow strong.
I hope that each of you is able to fulfill a part in the other that has not yet been filled.
And that by fulfilling each other, your marriage will be full with love.
May each of you always be able to add to the other's enjoyment of life,
As you create a new family that will always be a part of my own.

Reprinted with permission.

That Jay could express his thoughts more thoroughly through e-mail than in spontaneous conversations was an observation that Jay first noted independently. Because e-mail allowed him the time to choose his words with care, Jay believed that he had found a medium through which to communicate the words that he experienced difficulty generating in verbal conversations with others. Consequently, Jay was able to use e-mail to re-enter his role as an older brother in ways that he had previously been unable to.

> Like the last e-mail I wrote to my sister [see Figure 5.3]. She was having a hard time, she just moved, and she's getting ready for the wedding and her fiancée's mother, I think she's [fiancée's mother] really sick. And I tried to be her older brother, you know, to help her. I wanted to help her if I could. And I think that what I said in the [e-mail] letter I probably couldn't have said it all just talking to her. The words just wouldn't have come fast enough. We would have ended the phone call before I could have thought of it. But I said those things in my e-mail to her. I said things older brothers say. Maybe that sounds stupid but it meant a lot to me to act like her older brother.

Similarly, through e-mail, Jay embarked upon the creation of an extended family of individuals who demonstrated sincere interest in his well-being. For example, through e-mail, Jay began to correspond

FIGURE 5.3. Jay's E-Mail to His Sister Illustrating His Ability to Convey His Thoughts More Articulately in Written Words

Dear Sarah:

I hope that Andrew's mom is feeling more hopeful and better and maintaining positive thinking. I hope you're finding healthy ways to deal with the natural stresses of moving, getting married, and caring for Andrew's mother's ill health. I'm sending you my love and support to deal with your new life with all of its pressures and pleasures. I have confidence in your ability to handle all these new situations well.

As for my birthday, I don't want a present. Seeing you will be a great and meaningful present.

I love you very much.

Jay

Reprinted with permission.

with the president of the college that he had attended at the time of his injury. This college president had maintained contact with Jay's mother throughout Jay's acute and post-acute rehabilitation periods; she had consistently sent Jay cards and letters throughout the past years to express her continued interest and concern. Until Jay began his participation in the intervention, his mother had replied to all of the college president's inquiries, relaying information about Jay's progress without Jay's actual input. When Jay was introduced to his adapted e-mail program, he assumed responsibility for replying to his own mail and began to personally correspond with the college president directly.

Jay's "New Family"

Additionally, Jay attempted to develop extended-family relationships with two other men–a male client who resided at a different facility group home and a male direct-care staff member employed by the TBI facility. Because as a child and adolescent, Jay did not have access to positive male figures in his life, I believed that Jay would benefit from the opportunity to create extended-family big-brother relationships. These three men–Jay, the male client, and the direct-care staff member–regularly began to engage in activities that could support the resumption of post-injury adult male gender roles (e.g., attending sporting events, visiting jazz clubs, and dining out in community restaurants). The older male client, Jack, was Jay's first friend at the TBI rehabilitation facility and may have been one of the first adult friends Jay had made since injury. Although they did not share similar cultural backgrounds, Jack was able to stimulate Jay's intellect and thus provided ample opportunity for Jay to learn the skills of conversational banter. In the culture of the TBI rehabilitation facility, Jack was well known as a gregarious and engaging individual whose friendship was sought by many clients. His extension of friendship to Jay encouraged clients who had previously ostracized Jay to view him more favorably. Because Jack was able to model the skills of sociability and affability, he inadvertently provided Jay with the opportunity to learn the skills needed to form and maintain friendships. Jay began to mirror Jack's personable interaction style and soon developed a larger repertoire of social behaviors. Simultaneously, we (myself and the rehabilitation counselor, Eric) challenged Jay to obtain social interaction skills through role-playing and practice with others in the facility and community setting.

Jay's Home Environment: Resolving Conflict

Jay expressed particular concern that he had not established positive relationships with his fellow community group home members. The conflicted relationships that Jay had developed with the individuals sharing his community residence reminded him uncomfortably of his childhood home life. For Jay, the re-experience of a combative home environment caused him to feel pessimistic about his ability to create more satisfying relationships as an adult. Again, we challenged Jay to develop more positive patterns of interaction with the individuals sharing his group home by role-playing (in one-to-one sessions) specific negative situations that had actually occurred. During these role-playing sessions, Jay was encouraged to generate and practice alternative responses that would serve to establish more harmonious relationships. We also helped Jay to better understand how his own patterns of behavior contributed to confrontation. In several sessions, Jay and the group home members with whom he shared the greatest friction expressed their grievances face-to-face with mediation from either myself or Eric. These sessions provided Jay and his housemates with greater understanding of each individual's perceptions and personal needs. Several of Jay's fellow group home members expressed a lack of understanding regarding Jay's OCD and stated their belief that Jay acted intentionally to disrupt the home environment. Education regarding the nature of OCD and reassurance from Jay that he was not intentionally causing others strife, served to decrease the level of animosity between Jay and his roommates.

> I feel for the first time that I'm more accepted here. I don't feel like everyone hates me anymore. That means so much to me because I always wanted to have friends like normal people. . . . So it means a lot that I can finally feel at peace in my own home. And it means a lot that I can actually do something good about maintaining the peace.

Mentors, Role Models, and Father-Figures

Because of Jay's poor pre-morbid relationships with the adult males in his life, it became particularly important to provide him with the opportunity to develop a mentor-protégé relationship with a same-gender health professional. The individual who agreed to develop a mentoring relationship with Jay was the facility's neuropsychologist. The neuropsychologist, Dr. Murphy, was an adult male in his forties who had initially completed a battery of neuropsychological tests for Jay's admission but had not provided treatment. The two men began to meet weekly, not for formal psychological sessions but rather to engage in joint activities that would afford Jay the opportunity to develop a relationship with an adult male mentor or surrogate coach/teacher. Activities engaged in included fishing, attending baseball games, visiting coffee houses, and browsing in bookstores. During each of their sessions, Jay and his male mentor, Dr. Murphy, discussed Jay's concerns about creating meaningful work, developing friendships, and engaging in dating relationships. Having access to a caring and accepting adult male with whom to discuss his concerns was a novel experience for Jay.

> Dr. Murphy is someone I consider to be a close friend. He's someone I can confide in; I trust him. . . . I never really trusted any adults when I was younger. And I didn't have any older brothers or father-figures to help me out, or you know, pave the way for me so to speak.

The Need to Practice Pre-Dating Skills

Jay also desired to assume a dating role. Because he had not engaged in dating relationships extensively prior to his injury, Jay had not developed the social skills necessary for interacting with women in a social context. It is likely, too, that Jay's neurologic injury may have compounded the existence of poor pre-morbid social skills. At this stage in Jay's rehabilitation course, he needed to develop pre-dating skills–or skills that would allow him to comfortably interact with females in the context of platonic relationships. Over several sessions I role-played use of pre-dating skills with Jay until he was able to consistently demonstrate appropriate social interaction skills without cueing. At that time, I arranged for Jay to increase his interaction with female clients in community settings. For example, on several occasions, Jay and a female client ate dinner together in a community restaurant. During these sessions, I was present to assist Jay with such skills as establishing appropriate eye contact and personal space, initiating and responding to conversational topics, and maintaining an appropriate pattern of interaction based on turn-taking.

I feel I can talk to women much more easily now. I used to say dumb things or not know what to say at all. But now I feel better about just going up to someone I've seen around the [sheltered] workshop or the campus and saying hi to her.

JAY: THE ADAPTATION OF ACTIVITIES THAT SUPPORTED THE ACQUISITION OF MALE GENDER ROLES (TIER 2)

It was important to assist Jay in the adaptation of several pre-injury activities for post-injury participation (in accordance with existing sequelae secondary to Jay's neurologic injury). One of Jay's most personally meaningful activities that required adaptation for post-injury participation was that of writing. As noted, Jay was required to change his hand dominance post-injury from left to right as a result of left upper extremity spasticity. Writing with his right hand, however, was awkward and did not allow Jay to record his thoughts quickly enough before his short-term memory deficits interfered with recall. Jay was fortunate in that his mother offered him the use of her computer until she was able to purchase one for his own personal use.

Because Jay possessed a left hemianopsia (visual field cut) the computer keyboard and screen were positioned just right of midline to accommodate his visual deficits. The left edge of the computer screen was highlighted with red tape to enhance Jay's visual attendance to information displayed on the left side of the screen. Similarly, to decrease the visual complexity of the keyboard, specific commonly used keys were highlighted (i.e., tab indent, cap lock, backspace, delete) for easier visual identification.

Jay's computer program was also modified to increase his ability to use his word processing and e-mail programs independently. Options listed on the initial main menu screen were reduced to three icons: word processing, weekly schedule, and e-mail. Within each of these programs, tool bar options were similarly decreased to display only main functions (e.g., file open/close, save/save as, print, exit). For example, Jay's e-mail program was redesigned to allow him to readily view current messages as soon as he clicked on the e-mail icon. At the end of a message a screen prompt asked if he wished to reply to sender. The e-mail tool bar was recreated to display the e-mail addresses that Jay most frequently used. Clicking on a particular address enabled Jay to compose and send a letter without worrying about the need to access address files.

Similarly, Jay's computer scheduling program allowed him to view his weekly schedule by clicking on the schedule icon. Appointments could be easily recorded and deleted by clicking on the time slot and typing in the necessary information. Jay's schedule program was used to help him to organize and implement a weekly array of adult male gender activities that he personally chose. By possessing ready access to his weekly schedule, Jay was able to assess if he had made arrangements to occupy his free hours with activities that would allow him to engage in adult male gender roles. In this way, Jay was encouraged to assume the adult responsibility of planning his own schedule rather than relying on staff to organize his activities (other than scheduled therapies). The ability to independently organize a schedule of self-chosen adult activities enhanced Jay's sense of personal causation. While Jay continued to require staff assistance for transportation and money management, he did not report the sense of lost life control that he verbalized at the outset of his occupational therapy intervention.

> I still don't feel totally autonomous living here [in the community group home] but I can see where I can exercise adult control over my own pursuits and things I'd like to do. It makes me feel more in control, like a responsible adult.

RUDY: WRESTLING WITH SEXUAL DISINHIBITION. THE REBUILDING OF ADULT MALE GENDER ROLES (TIER 1)

One of Rudy's most disturbing role losses after injury concerned his inability to resume a dating/courtship role. Prior to his accident, Rudy had enjoyed an active social life that included a series of monogamous sexual relationships with women. At 23 years of age, the time of his injury, Rudy was actively indulging his adult independence and recent return from Vietnam.

His injury occurred to the dorsolateral frontal cortex and hypothalamic regions–areas that play a role in regulating sexual desire and response (Geschwind & Galaburda, 1987). It was likely that as a result of neurologic insult to these structures, Rudy became sexually disinhibited and began to exhibit inappropriate behaviors with women in public settings. Because of his sexual disinhibition, Rudy's placement in TBI residential programs may have become problematic and consequently, Rudy experienced a series of admissions and discharges from various residential facilities. Discharges often occurred in response to a specific event in which the facility could no longer tolerate Rudy's sexually inappropriate behaviors.

In the first two years of Rudy's current residential placement, a similar situation occurred in which Rudy became sexually and physically aggressive with a female client whom he was attempting to date. Rather than discharge Rudy from the facility, however, the treatment team physically separated Rudy from female clients by moving him to an all-male group home and restricting his community access.

It is important to note also that at age 40–while Rudy was residing in a supportive living arrangement in Florida–he discharged himself against his family's wishes to marry a woman who, shortly after, stole the remaining money left from his insurance settlement. This failed marriage left Rudy feeling betrayed and unable to achieve an adult male spousal role.

Dating: Rudy's Foremost Priority

When Rudy volunteered to participate in the present study, he identified his wish to engage in dating relationships as his foremost priority. Like Jay, Rudy needed to develop a repertoire of pre-dating skills in order to interact with women in more appropriate ways. Initially Rudy and I compiled a list of the socially inappropriate behaviors that he displayed in public. These included prolonged staring, violating social norms of personal space, frequently touching others' shoulders and arms, and verbalizing sexual propositions. Rudy was aware that he exhibited these behaviors and that they were considered to be inappropriate. Rudy and I then discussed how to replace these behaviors with more socially acceptable ones. To identify appropriate interaction skills with women, Rudy and I observed men and women in the larger community environment (e.g., at shopping centers and malls, in restaurants, and at the bank). During these observation sessions, appropriate eye contact, respect of another's personal space, and appropriate conversational topics were noted. Rudy and I began to role-play use of appropriate interaction skills, first within the safety of the clinic, and then within the actual community setting. Feedback regarding Rudy's use of skills was offered after each session.

After one month, Rudy began to consistently demonstrate more socially appropriate behaviors in role-playing sessions with me. At this time, he then began to test his skills within the context of dating situations with female clients at the facility. During these sessions, either I or Eric accompanied Rudy while he joined female companions for dinner in community restaurants, shopping at the mall, and walking in a local park. I was present on these occasions to cue Rudy when his behaviors deviated from those he had learned in his role-playing sessions. As Rudy more consistently demonstrated that he required less supervision from me, he was then given permission from his facility treatment team to accompany a female client to dinner in a community restaurant. During these dinners, it was agreed by Rudy and his treatment team members that a therapist (either myself or Eric) would be seated at a nearby table in order to offer distant supervision. In this way, Rudy had achieved a greater degree of privacy and autonomy in dating relationships than that which he had previously been afforded within his rehabilitation facility.

Rudy's treatment team members had not attempted to offer him social skill training in the context of dating relationships–instead attempting to deal with Rudy's inappropriate behaviors by restricting his access to women. By allowing Rudy to practice social interaction with women in progressively less supervised settings, Rudy was able to demonstrate that he could assume more socially acceptable behaviors. However, because of the nature of Rudy's neurologic injury, he will likely continue to struggle with some degree of sexual disinhibition–particularly inappropriate verbalizations regarding sexual activity. Fortunately, Rudy's treatment team members have agreed to continue to allow him to engage in dating activities with women in supervised settings. It is likely that the ability to actively engage in dating relationships has contributed to Rudy's decreased obsessive-like verbalizations regarding participation in a romantic relationship.

However, Rudy has not as yet met a female who wishes to share a sexual relationship with him and he continues to readily verbalize his need for physical stimulation. To alleviate what is likely a neurologically driven need for heightened sexual stimulation, Rudy has begun to use the services of a licensed massage therapist when he is able to save money sufficient for the therapist's fee. While body massage does not mitigate Rudy's desire for orgasmic activity, he does report that it lessens his need to be touched by another human in a compassionate way.

You know, when you're a client with a head injury, no one
touches you except in a clinical way–like you're a specimen or
something. No one hugs you or kisses you. I haven't been
touched by another human being in a loving way since my accident. It makes me feel less than human, less than a dog even. At
least a dog gets a pat on the head every once in awhile. Getting a
body massage makes me feel more human again, more in touch
with my humanness and manliness.

Male Camaraderie

At the intervention's outset, Rudy also verbalized disappointment
regarding his lost role as a male friend and cited as a primary goal his
desire to rebuild a circle of male friends with whom he could share a
sense of camaraderie. Because Rudy was now in his late 40s, he felt
generationally and emotionally distanced from most of the other male
clients who–typical of TBI statistics–were 20 to 30 years old. At the
same time, Rudy reported that he did not feel close to the male staff
members who shared his age group as a result of the professional
distance preserved between client and staff. Essentially, Rudy felt
alone in his experience of head injury and lacked opportunities to talk
with other men who could express empathy from similar personal
experience. Eric introduced Rudy to an older male client in his 50s
who resided in a main facility campus unit due to severe physical
deficits secondary to TBI. Like Rudy, this male client came from a
traditional Italian-American background, served in the Vietnam war,
had been married and divorced, and experienced role losses similar to
those of Rudy's (e.g., husband, sexual partner, friend, worker). This
relationship provided both men access to a male confidant with whom
to share a sense of affinity.

[Male client's name] and I share a similar life experience and
mental knowledge of what it's like to be a 50 year old man with a
head injury; to have lived life on this earth for twenty-some years
with a head injury that changed my adult life and life choices in
ways you can't imagine–ways I couldn't even imagine if it didn't
happen to me. It feels great to talk to someone who understands
what I'm talking about. . . . I don't feel so much like the odd ball
from Mars with [client's name].

Mentoring Other Clients

With Eric's help, Rudy also initiated a friendship with a younger male client who shared his group home residence. This male client was legally blind and, as a result of a left upper and lower extremity hemiparesis (muscular weakness), required assistance to negotiate steps, curb cuts, and unlevel surface transitions. Because Rudy expressed an interest in offering assistance to this client, Eric taught Rudy how to offer minimal physical aid under the direct supervision of a staff member. It is curious that while Rudy and this particular housemate shared a residence, they rarely interacted–a phenomenon that appeared common amongst many of the community group home residents. Most interactions initiated by clients were directed toward staff members–a situation that may have been characteristic of the cultural norms of the TBI rehabilitation facility. Clients may have been encouraged to communicate primarily with direct care staff in order to ensure greater staff control of group home life. However, encouraging communication primarily with staff members did not allow Rudy to build friendships with the other men who shared his home; it became apparent that in order to help Rudy to rebuild friendships, the pattern of communication used in the group homes needed to be readjusted. Helping Rudy to interact directly with the male client who was legally blind became one way to reintroduce Rudy to the skills necessary for rebuilding male friendships.

Perhaps because Rudy neither possessed a younger brother nor experienced a positive relationship with his own older brother, he became interested in the idea of creating an extended-family big-brother relationship with the younger male client who was visually impaired.

> I feel that with my years of wisdom, being the man that I am, I can contribute to someone else's situation. I'd like to use my twenty-some years of head injury experience to help someone else who–God bless em–hasn't lived with a head injury as long as I have. Someone I could take under my wing and show em the ropes so to speak.

When Rudy went shopping in the community (accompanied by a staff member), he would purchase and bring home small items in an effort to enhance the younger man's quality of life (e.g., coffee and donuts). He'd make himself available to the younger man for what he called "man-to-man talks" and offered encouraging words in passing (e.g., "you're doing a great job; keep up the good work"). It appeared that Rudy was attempting to recreate his role as the older male guide he had often desired but never actually encountered.

> [Younger male client's name] is a great kid. He's like a younger brother or nephew to me. It makes me feel like a first rate man to help him. Like I'm doing something for his good. I'd like to be for him the older, wiser man he can go to if he needs help from a man who's been around the block a couple of times or more.

The Longed-For Male Mentor

The older wiser male mentor became a commonly verbalized theme for Rudy. Often he expressed regret that he had not found an older brother-surrogate figure who could both understand his experience of head injury and guide his life journey. In all of Rudy's facility rehabilitation placements, he had always been one of the oldest, male clients, having sustained his injury in the early 1970s–a time when the medical profession had little effective emergency care techniques for individuals sustaining brain injury (Miller, 1993). It is a reflection of Rudy's perseverance and life vitality that he even survived his automobile accident at a time when medical procedures offered minimal hope. Long-term treatment of individuals with head injury did not become readily available until the early 1980s. Until that time, individuals who sustained TBI–those who survived–were left to forge their own rehabilitation paths with little resources (Miller, 1990).

In an attempt to accommodate Rudy's desire for a male mentor, Eric invited Rudy to develop a mentor-protégé relationship with him. Eric was a man in his mid-forties who had worked in TBI rehabilitation for over 10 years. While Eric possessed intimate knowledge of Rudy through case management functions, he had not engaged in one-to-one activities with him. Over the course of the four-month intervention period, Rudy and Eric came to develop their own male rituals; for example, their "fireside chats" in which both men would convene for an hour of each day in a private den flanked by a huge stone fireplace–hence the name, "fireside chat." Together, Rudy and his mentor, Eric, attended hobby conventions, drag races, and day trips to Atlantic City and the racetrack. It is a reflection of Rudy and Eric's achieved level of joint understanding that they created their own set of words describing the head injury experience.

I finally found the man I've been looking for to model myself after his image and intelligence for the last 20 years. Eric understands me to a tee. He knows exactly what I'm trying to say when I'm trying to describe what it's like for me in some such situation because of this head injury.

I feel completely accepted by Eric. He doesn't look at me like I'm from another planet–like so many other people do. . . . When I have a problem he's the first one I turn to cause I know he'll impart his advice and it will be advice that I can use that will benefit myself.

Giving Something Back to the Community

Eric was also instrumental in helping Rudy to rebuild community member roles. After Rudy's accident, he could neither find employment that was personally meaningful nor that offered a salary commensurate with his pay as a longshoreman. In Rudy's current facility placement, he had refused to engage in the piecework offered by the facility's sheltered workshop as a standard component of all client programming. Consequently, Rudy–not able to rebuild a satisfactory work role–spent many daytime hours sleeping or watching television.

As mentioned, Rudy grew up in an Italian-American family who cultivated their own garden vegetables and prepared homegrown cuisine. Because Rudy often enthusiastically described his childhood memories of tending his family's garden, his mentor, Eric, believed that planting and tending a community garden could offer Rudy an opportunity to participate in meaningful work through which he could contribute to others.

I can't tell you how happy I am to get down on my hands and knees in the dirt and tend a living plant that I know, is only gonna survive if I take care of it. It's in my Italian-American blood to grow and cook vegetables. I feel like I was meant to be doing this kinda work, ya know what I mean? It's in me since I'm a kid. It's me expressing a deep part of me.

It's a wonderful thing to grow something with your own sweat and blood that's actually appreciated by others. When me and [staff member's name] cook my tomatoes down into a sauce and we eat it with spaghetti or have 'em in a salad for dinner, I feel great. Like the whole world is smiling cause of something I did–instead of some dumb doofus thing I did, which is usually more the case.

In Rudy's cultural value system, the act of food preparation and meal consumption provided social avenues through which to form and maintain intimate relationships. Invitations to share a meal were used as vehicles to strengthen social ties. By providing an opportunity to participate in a central component of meal preparation, Rudy was able to engage in a social activity that was both congruent with his cultural values and served to contribute to others' physical welfare and health.

The idea of contributing to others through work emerged repeatedly in Rudy's conversations concerning the loss of his work role. He frequently verbalized an interest in volunteering his time to educate others about TBI, substance use, and hypersexuality after neurologic insult. Rudy received the chance to impart his knowledge to others when I asked him to speak to a class of occupational therapy students concerning his experience of living with a head injury. This was an opportunity for Rudy to assume the role of expert–a role that seemed to continuously evade his grasp as a client.

> Speaking to the students gave me a chance to impart the knowl-edge I've acquired as a forty-some year old man with head injury to others. It made me feel like, yeah, I do have something of importance to say that will help other people. I felt like the wise man I know myself to be deep inside. It made me feel important, like people valued what I could say about living with a head injury for twenty-some years.

Education had gained considerable importance to Rudy after his injury. As a 23 year old man who had completed high school and returned from Vietnam, Rudy had not been interested in furthering his education during the period just prior to his injury. But in the years since, Rudy began to regret that he had not been able to assume the role of student/adult learner and frequently verbalized his desire to return to school. In the last two years, Rudy recognized that he pos-sessed natural artistic talents–a discovery that occurred through expo-sure to painting during his recreational therapy sessions. As a child, Rudy remembered drawing but receiving no exceptional praise for his work. Because painting and drawing were not valued activities in his family system, Rudy instead pursued competitive sports and athletics.

With some assistance from Eric, Rudy became involved in a ceramics class sponsored by a local community college. Rudy also requested that his extended-family little brother attend with him.

> I feel like I'm doing something with my mind and my hands instead of just sitting around [name of facility]. I'm doing something to increase my mental stimulation. . . . It feels good to be amongst other people who are just as interested in improving their knowledge and experience and lot in life like I am.

> And to go with [extended-family little brother's name] makes it all the sweeter. This is an opportunity for him and me to bond in a man-to-man sort of way such that I can feel like the older man giving a hand to the younger man. And that makes me feel like I can impart my knowledge and use my experience to act of assistance to someone else.

Rudy also began to use his artwork as a vehicle through which to contribute to his family members. In the years since his injury, Rudy had been particularly concerned that he had accepted a wealth of generosity and assistance from his family members without being able to reciprocate–a situation that for him wounded his identity as an independent man able to provide for his loved ones. In the past 20 years, Rudy's sole role within his family system had become that of care recipient rather than provider. He perceived himself to be a burden upon his elderly, ill father and felt responsible for thrusting a caregiving role upon both of his parents and brother. Rudy began to assume a more active avuncular role with his nephews and nieces by using his artistic talent to create painted wooden toys and beaded jewelry for them (as described below). These endeavors helped Rudy to participate in his familial role as a caregiver, rather than only a care recipient–a role that helped Rudy to alter his perceived status within the family hierarchy.

> Now I'm actually giving something back to my family through the younger generation of [family's surname]. I always saw myself as the generous Italian-American uncle who could give my nieces and nephews my knowledge or you know, slip them a five [dollar bill] now and then. And now I'm making them toys and

such and my niece, she just loves the necklaces; she eats them up. She calls me and says, "Uncle Rudy, when are ya gonna make me another necklace?" And I say, "Honey, just put in your order." It makes me feel a real part of the family in a good way. You know, not just asking for help all the time. I wanna be able to give something back.

RUDY: THE PARTICIPATION IN ACTIVITIES THAT SUPPORTED THE ACQUISITION OF MALE GENDER ROLES (TIER 2)

Activities in which Rudy engaged prior to his participation in the intervention largely supported his role as a client in a TBI rehabilitation facility but did not facilitate his role as an adult man. Rudy articulated this irony clearly when he stated,

If you're a good client and do your chores and go to work and eat your dinner and take a piss when they tell you to and don't cause no trouble, then you end up without any sense of yourself as an adult man. What kinda rehabilitation is that?

The activities that supported Rudy's role of a client were incongruent with his desire to assume the role of an adult man. When the intervention began, Rudy urgently wanted to engage in dating activities but was prohibited by his treatment team members due to past indiscretions. Rather than attempting to assist Rudy to attain more appropriate social skills, however, his treatment team members restricted Rudy's access to women both within the facility and larger community. The activities that Rudy self-initiated to resume a dating role consisted of perusing newspaper personal ads and watching X-rated films alone in his room–both activities that facilitated further isolation. Helping Rudy to resume dating activities with supervision was a considerable gain toward the resumption of desired male roles.

Rebelling Against Communication Restrictions: Reaching Out to Others

Similarly, Rudy's phone and community travel restrictions–imposed by the TBI facility–prevented him from more fully engaging in friend roles. These restrictions prevented Rudy from calling friends and arranging social activities. For example, while Rudy had become friends with a male client residing at a main campus unit, he was initially unable to call this man or to visit without arranging for staff accompaniment. Rudy and Eric attempted to demonstrate to Rudy's treatment team members that he would not abuse facility phone privileges if permitted an allotted sum of phone calls. Through the creation of a weekly schedule of phone calls to specific individuals, Rudy proposed to his treatment team members that he required phone privileges to maintain relationships and arrange social activities in order to support his role as an adult man. On a trial basis, Rudy was permitted three 10 minute local phone calls per week. Each successful phone contact was recorded on a check-off sheet to cue Rudy's recall of which friends he had established contact with and which were not available to answer his call. Using the weekly phone schedule, Rudy was able to demonstrate to his treatment team members that he could responsibly make an allotted number of phone calls in order to maintain the meaningful relationships and activities that supported his role as an adult friend, extended-family member, and individual involved in dating/courtship relationships.

Physically arranging visits with friends and dates with female companions was more difficult. Due to staffing shortages, Rudy was often unable to find a direct-care staff available to accompany him to other facility residences or to supervise community outings with female dates. Occasionally Rudy independently secured transportation on the facility van as it passed by his group home en route to either the main facility campus, apartments, or other group homes.

Gardening, toy and jewelry making, and public speaking were all activities that supported the rebuilding of Rudy's community member and familial roles. These activities required adaptation, however, in order to enable Rudy's independent participation. Gardening activities were simplified into three components–initial planting, daily watering, and harvesting of vegetables. Tomato plants were chosen as the primary vegetable due to their hardiness and requirement for minimal care. The use of already grown starter plants simplified the task by reducing the need to seed. Rudy helped plant ten starter tomato stalks in the backyard of his group home. Again, use of a daily watering schedule was implemented for Rudy to follow independently. When the tomato plants grew tall, a staff member accompanied Rudy to the store to purchase wood and string and taught Rudy how to secure the plant stems to the stakes. Rudy was also required to pick all of the tomatoes upon ripening and distribute excess tomatoes to nearby community group homes (under the supervision of a staff member).

Similarly, toy and jewelry making were simplified by purchasing wooden kits of trains, trucks, and boxes that Rudy glued together and painted. Instructions for toy construction were rewritten in simplified 4-5 step directions, thus enabling Rudy to create the toys independently. Likewise, Rudy made his own necklaces by molding beads out of pre-colored self-hardening sculpting material that could be purchased in a variety of colors.

Rudy's public speaking engagement was also modified to facilitate his experience of success. Prior to his guest lecture, Rudy and I met to outline the topics that he wished to present to his audience of students. We agreed that specific topics would be discussed in a question and answer format so that Rudy would not be responsible for independently following an established lecture outline. Instead, I cued Rudy throughout the lecture by asking him questions that he had previously chosen to address. In this way, Rudy appeared to conduct his lecture effortlessly, answering questions with the seeming ease of an experienced public speaker.

ED: NO LONGER MOTHER'S LITTLE BOY.
THE REBUILDING OF ADULT MALE
GENDER ROLES (TIER 1)

One important component of the intervention concerned helping the men to engage more fully in their roles as family members. Ed, however, reported that he had already established a close relationship with his mother, receiving daily phone contact and visiting every weekend at her home. Ed experienced conflicting dual emotions for his mother. While he enjoyed the nurturance and care that his mother was able to provide, he also felt infantalized by and dependent upon her protection–emotions that were discordant with his desire to become an independent man.

> I love my mother. She's been there for me in the darkest hours. But sometimes she babies me too. I love her. I don't want to hurt her.

The emotional bind of wanting to continue to receive his mother's affection but to lessen his dependence upon her, likely caused Ed to feel confused and guilty. Ed barely possessed the skills to articulate his emotional bind; the high-level problem-solving skills necessary to actually resolve his conflicting emotions for his mother were beyond Ed's present psychosocial abilities.

By having the opportunity to go home every weekend, Ed escaped the social task of learning the skills necessary to build friendships. Because his weekends were also planned by his mother, Ed was similarly relieved from having to arrange an array of social activities sufficient to occupy his non-workday hours. While Ed verbally expressed a desire to build friendships and engage in social activities, he may have also experienced anxiety when confronted with the challenge of learning new social skills. Consequently, Ed–not possessing the skills to build the relationships he desired as an adult man–opted to spend weekends with his mother.

Because Ed's only close pre-injury female relationship had been the one he shared with his mother, we speculated that Ed might benefit from a surrogate big-sister relationship with a female client also residing at the TBI rehabilitation facility. It was reasoned that Ed would benefit most from interaction with a female who could treat him with the care and concern of a younger brother while still providing the opportunity to practice social skills with a female other than his mother. Through his employment at the sheltered workshop, Ed had encountered a female client named Lyn with whom he had never spoken. Lyn, a divorced woman in her late 40s with two adult children, resided in a 24 hour supervised main facility campus unit due to intermittent seizure activity. I asked Lyn if she would consider assuming a big-brother role with Ed on a trial basis. I explained that becoming a surrogate big-sister would involve spending one-to-one time with Ed in order to help him to acquire greater social skills with women.

Perhaps because Lyn felt that she had missed her own children's transition into adulthood as a result of her TBI, she generously welcomed the opportunity to become a surrogate big-sister to Ed. Challenging Ed's shyness and discomfort interacting with women was easy for Lyn, as she was both extroverted and gregarious, and readily engaged Ed in conversation that required him to respond appropriately and maintain eye contact. Because initiating conversation was more difficult for Ed, he and I began to role-play conversations in which he could practice the skills necessary to independently enter a conversation and broach a new topic area. Ed then began to practice initiating conversations with Lyn while I observed to offer assistance and later feedback.

In the workshop, Lyn regularly greeted Ed and began to join him for lunch in the facility's cafeteria–a marked change in Ed's previous pattern of isolative behavior. Because Lyn was well liked and had several friends at the facility, she was further able to expose Ed to increased socialization by inviting others to share the lunch period with them. When we became aware that Ed had gone from eating alone to sharing lunch with a group of people in a relatively short period of time, Eric and I began to alternately join the lunch group to assist Ed with group interaction skills. Initiating conversation in a dyad was a novel and difficult experience for Ed; speaking up spontaneously in a group was likely frightening and anxiety provoking. In the complexity of group interaction, Ed became lost and deferred speaking to other group members.

While Ed's exposure to increased socialization was positive, I had not intended for Ed to confront the challenge of group skills until he had grown comfortable with dyadic interaction. To help Ed learn to initiate conversation and contribute spontaneous verbalizations in a group discussion, I began to role-play use of these skills with Ed and another male client. Verbal skills learned in role-playing sessions were then practiced in the lunch group with supervision from either Eric or myself. After two months, Ed was able to maintain eye contact with other group members, appropriately respond to direct questions, and contribute spontaneous verbalizations to already established group conversations. Initiating a new topic of discussion, however, continued to present a challenge to Ed.

In his one-to-one time spent with Lyn, however, Ed had begun to grow more comfortable initiating his own areas of topic interest. Staff members employed in the vocational workshop also reported that Ed had become more friendly and commonly greeted other clients–rather than only speaking to staff as was Ed's previous communication pattern.

> I like people. I'm a people person. But it was never easy for me to talk to people–even before my accident. It's still hard. But I can talk more now. I can say hello and how are you. And people talk more to me now too.

The Men's Group

While Ed had begun to learn the skills of social interaction, he had not as yet begun to use those skills to form deeper friendships. Eric and I believed that it would be beneficial to provide the opportunity for Ed to participate in a men's group comprised of similar others. Because no such group existed, Eric created one by inviting three other male clients and Ed to convene weekly for discussion and community outings. Because the three male clients who joined the group were not particularly gregarious, Ed may have felt less threatened socially and thus initiated conversation more readily. Two of the men who joined the group used to share a community group home residence with Ed but had since moved to the apartment program. Interestingly, while Ed did not form relationships with these men when they shared a residence, he now expressed interest in visiting at their new apartments. Unwittingly, Eric had invited men to join the group who had become role models for Ed–clients who used to occupy Ed's social position within the rehabilitation facility but who had achieved greater independent living.

> [Male client's names] are people I respect. They moved on. They used to be where I am but now they moved on to the apartments. It gives me hope that I can live in the apartments too.

While Ed spoke freely with these men during group meetings, he did not possess the skills to arrange social activities outside of the group. Ed and I role-played how to ask for phone numbers and inquire whether others would like to meet for dinner or a game of cards. Because Ed did not possess the same phone and community travel restrictions that Rudy did, using the phone to contact friends and arrange social outings was not problematic. Instead, it was Ed's lack of phone skills and ability to initiate communication that presented primary challenges. Ed and I first generated a list of possible activities in which Ed could independently participate with his male friends (e.g., meeting for dinner at a local community restaurant, visiting at each others' residence for card games). We then role-played the skills needed to initiate telephone conversations and extend invitations for social get-togethers. When Ed felt comfortable role-playing these skills, he then began to practice making actual phone calls with cueing from me. On the first two occasions that Ed arranged to meet a male friend for dinner at a nearby community restaurant (located within walking distance), I attended to provide assistance with social interaction skills, community travel, and a repertoire of community skills that Ed did not commonly use–for example, menu reading, bill paying, and tipping.

Designing Activities to Enhance Social Initiation

Ed appeared to be gaining independence in the skills needed to form and maintain friendships. However, when I began to reduce my level of assistance and no longer accompanied Ed on community outings with friends, Ed's initiation of social contact began to wane. Ed's neurologic injury involved the orbitofrontal cortex, a region of the brain that regulates motivation and initiation of activity (Miller, 1993). Individuals who sustain injury to the orbitofrontal cortex commonly appear to lack motivation and demonstrate difficulty initiating activity despite a professed desire. Unfortunately, staff members–who may not understand the neurologic underpinnings of head injury seque-lae–often incorrectly assume that someone like Ed simply does not care to participate in available activities, and consequently no longer attempt to assist the individual with initiation. Ed had fallen victim to this misperception in the past when staff members in his group home misinterpreted Ed's poor initiation as a lack of desire and abandoned their attempts to enhance his participation in social events.

Individuals with orbitofrontal lobe damage, however, can sometimes carry out an activity independently if assisted with the initial stages of performance (Miller, 1993). In Ed's case, a minimal amount of staff cueing was required to assist him with the initiation of both phone calls and visits to friends at pre-arranged times. A written phone schedule was introduced to cue Ed to maintain contact with both his surrogate big-sister and the two individuals from the men's group with whom he had begun to establish friendships. Similarly, Ed was also presented with a weekly schedule planner and was encouraged to choose one evening per week to arrange a social activity (unaccompanied by staff). A direct-care staff member, Bob, who worked in Ed's group home began to assume responsibility for weekly schedule planning with Ed and regularly cued him to maintain his schedule of phone calls and community outings with friends. With this level of regular staff assis-tance, Ed was able to maintain his weekly social contact with the two men in the apartment program and with his surrogate big-sister.

The Appearance of a Surrogate Big-Brother

While Ed was beginning to rebuild his role as a friend, he continued to lack a relationship in which he could benefit from the guidance and concern bestowed by a surrogate big-brother or mentor. As mentioned, Ed did not experience positive pre-morbid relationships with the males in his life, feeling alienated from both his stepfather and brothers. At Ed's present rehabilitation facility, he was considered to be an unproblematic client–that is, a client who followed his prescribed programming without causing difficulty to staff and other residents. Ironically, Ed's compliance may have been related to his orbitofrontal lobe injury, causing him to appear well mannered and complaisant. An unproblematic client can sometimes receive less attention than needed, as staff members' focus tends to shift toward clients whose behavior warrants immediate response. Conversely, the affability and willingness to comply–characteristic of unproblematic clients–can also elicit increased staff member favors and affection. Fortunately, such was the case with Ed. Bob, the male direct-care staff member who assisted with Ed's weekly social planning, had demonstrated a fondness for Ed and, when the intervention began, expressed a desire to become Ed's surrogate big-brother/mentor. To facilitate this relationship, Bob was relieved from several residential duties to spend more one-to-one time with Ed.

> Bob has been a good friend to me. I can talk to him like a friend, like the friends I used to have in high school. We [Bob and Ed] go to [ball] games together and to 7-Eleven [quick serve store] for coffee. He helps me with things around the house. Like my schedule and making phone calls. I appreciate his help. He never says he's busy. He's always willing to help.

Developing Dating Skills

Like the other three men, Ed also desired to assume dating/courtship roles. However, because Ed had not participated in romantic relationships pre-injury, he lacked the most elemental skills needed to interact with women in a social context. Prior to his involvement in the intervention, Ed could barely maintain eye contact with females, let alone initiate a conversation and extend a social invitation. Ed's interaction with his surrogate big-sister, Lyn, helped to mitigate some of his shyness with women. However, the social skills Ed learned with

Lyn were those appropriate for a platonic friendship, and Ed continued to experience significant difficulty approaching female clients he wished to know more intimately. In the past two years, Ed and his rehabilitation counselor had unsuccessfully attempted to use a dating service for individuals with disabilities. While Ed had paid his $25.00 membership fee to join the dating service, he failed to receive contact from interested females–an occurrence that caused him to feel undesirable. The women at his current rehabilitation placement reportedly considered Ed to be more of an unsophisticated little brother rather than an adult man with whom to form a romantic bond. Much like the norms of high school dating, males in the TBI facility who were physically appealing, gregarious, and could successfully read and interpret social cues, were sought after as romantic partners.

Ed's lack of social adeptness with women was also beginning to disrupt his relationships with the other male clients who shared his group home–many of whom displayed a greater ease in the use of social skills with women. Ed, perhaps jealous of these other male's greater social skill proficiency, became argumentative in the home environment–particularly with one male client who had begun dating a female with whom Ed had been romantically interested.

First, Ed needed to obtain the skills necessary to express his emotions to women he wished to date. To decrease the level of difficulty inherent in speaking directly to women, we provided the opportunity for Ed to learn the skills of self-expression through letter writing. A particular female client, Arlene, who resided at the facility's twin site in an adjacent state was contacted by Eric to determine if she would like to establish a letter writing relationship with Ed. This particular female client previously resided at Ed's facility and knew of him; however, Ed could not remember her, perhaps because he shared neither a residence nor work site with her. The two began to regularly correspond with the assistance of Eric who helped Ed to compose and edit his letters. Subsequently, the activity of letter writing was added to Ed's weekly schedule of phone calls and visits with friends.

> I'm not seeing Arlene but we write every week. I like her and I know she likes me too. I feel like I have a girlfriend now. I'm happy. I wanted a girlfriend for a long time. . . . I'd like to see her. Maybe when Bob [direct-care staff/surrogate big-brother] takes me up there [to Arlene's residence].

In the second month of the intervention, as Ed became more comfortable expressing his thoughts through writing, Eric then began to assist Ed to transfer his communication skills to phone use. After several role-playing sessions in which Ed and Eric practiced the skills needed to call his female acquaintance, Ed began to make weekly phone calls to Arlene, first with cueing from Eric, and then independently. Interestingly, while Ed required cueing from a staff member to maintain his weekly phone contact with his two male friends, he independently remembered to call the woman he considered to be his girlfriend.

Expanding Community Member Roles

Additionally, with my assistance, Ed was able to obtain several community member roles. It was to Ed's credit that he had already re-established a work role that was personally satisfying; his employment at the facility's sheltered workshop afforded Ed at least one role through which he could rebuild his identity as an adult man.

> I like going to work–getting up every day and following a routine. It feels good to get done what I'm supposed to at work. I feel like I'm doing something with my life, like a responsible man.

Within the TBI facility, however, Ed's only other major role was that of a client. To allow Ed to assume a role in which he could contribute to the facility community, Bob (Ed's surrogate big-brother) helped him to become a part of the planning activities for the facility's Visitor's Day–an annual event in which family members are invited to join their loved ones for a fete-like summer festivity. At this event, therapists largely organize activities, run booths, and prepare and serve foods. Again, it is curious that the individuals residing at the site are not encouraged to assume greater involvement in the planning of activities. Instead the facility assumes a parental-like role–providing festivities for their clients rather than inviting them to be partners in the planning of events.

Ed and his surrogate big-brother manned the booth at which one attempts to lodge ping-pong balls into goldfish bowls. When Ed's mother first recognized Ed behind the booth at Visitor's Day, she instructed him to stop bothering the therapist, not understanding that he was actually helping to operate the booth. Ed's mother's response was likely elicited as a result of being unaccustomed to observing her son in an adult role. Ed, however, was ready to assume greater adult responsibilities.

> I felt proud. Everybody saw me running the booth at Visitor's Day. I was in charge for once. People came to me for help. I knew I could do it.

Bob also attempted to assist Ed to integrate more thoroughly into his role as a church member. As mentioned previously, while Ed had re-established his weekly Sunday church attendance after injury, he had neither met nor formed friendships with any of the other church members. With assistance from Bob, Ed began to sit amongst the congregation rather than off to the side in a special pew separating individuals with disabilities from other church members. This strategic seating change afforded Ed greater opportunity to meet his fellow church members and to begin to form acquaintances with individuals whom he regularly encountered. Ed learned the skills of introducing himself and greeting others through role-playing with Bob and me. At weekly Sunday services, Bob further assisted Ed with introductions and verbal greetings to other church members.

> I like church a lot better now. Now I know the people and they say hello to me. I feel more at home now. . . . Before I'd go and listen to the service and then go home. Now other people will say, "Hello. How are you?" And I say, "Hello. How are you? Nice to see you today." It's nice. I know that people like me now. One lady–she always wears a blue hat–she comes up to me and she shakes my hand and smiles. It's nice. I like it. It makes me feel good.

ED: "HOLD ON, I HAVE TO CHECK MY CALENDAR." THE PARTICIPATION IN ACTIVITIES THAT SUPPORTED THE ACQUISITION OF MALE GENDER ROLES (TIER 2)

Once Ed began to rebuild the relationships that supported his roles as friend, extended-family member, and individual involved in dating/courtship activities, he needed to assume the adult responsibility of organizing his participation in activities that would preserve his new roles (e.g., making phone calls, letter writing, and meeting others for dinner). Ed began to use an adapted weekly schedule planner with the assistance of Bob and myself. Initially Ed and I listed all of the new activities that he had recently assumed. Each activity's name was printed out on different colored stickers (e.g., phone call to John, letter to Arlene, dinner date with George). At the beginning of the week, Ed organized these stickers onto separate weekdays in order to arrange a balance of activities that would support his new adult male roles. As Ed introduced additional activities to his repertoire, new sticker labels were added to the weekly schedule planning activity. Initially Ed required assistance to both organize his weekly activities and follow through with participation. By the end of the intervention, Ed only required minimal cueing from a staff member to initiate his weekly schedule planning activity but could then implement the actual planning of activities independently. Assistance from a staff member was also needed to cue Ed to actually carry out the activities that he had chosen on each particular day. By teaching Ed to independently plan an array of weekly activities designed to support his adult male roles, Ed could readily observe how his own actions influenced his identity as an adult man.

> I feel more in control over my life. I'm doing things adults do. I am an adult. I have a social life like an adult man now. Before I didn't. I didn't have any friends. I didn't talk to people much.

Similarly, Ed's participation in letter writing was also adapted to allow him to build his skills of expression gradually. Initially, Eric helped Ed to begin each letter writing task by outlining several topics that Ed wished to address (e.g., expressing his happiness to have a friend with whom to write, describing his workweek). These topics were then re-ordered in accordance with Ed's weighting of importance. Essentially, Ed completed a letter by following the ordered outline of topic headings and elaborating upon each in a narrative format. Upon completion of a letter, Eric would then assist Ed with editing.

A Refresher Course in Community Travel Training

Likewise, Ed's planned dinners with friends were adapted to increase his independent participation. Fortunately, Ed's group home residence was located within walking distance of two inexpensive neighborhood restaurants. These local restaurants became a haven from the TBI facility for clients who had obtained independent travel status. It was in these restaurants that Ed and his two male friends often met for dinner. While Ed had obtained independence in community travel around his neighborhood, he had forgotten several of the walking routes as a result of failing to exercise his independent community travel privileges. Consequently, when Ed first arranged to meet one of his friends at a local restaurant, we realized that he had forgotten the correct route to follow. Several sessions of community travel training had to be re-implemented at that time to increase Ed's independence. Additionally, I practiced bill paying and tipping with Ed until he demonstrated the ability to calculate a check and make correct change independently. A pocket calculator and a wallet size card listing appropriate 15% and 20% tips for each dollar amount from one to 50 were also provided.

Using Cheat-Sheets at the Fair Booth

To adapt Ed's participation in operating the Goldfish Throw booth at Visitor's Day, the activity was divided into several components: collecting the three ticket stubs necessary to play, disbursing three ping-pong balls to the customer, retrieving stray balls from the ground, and alerting the supervising staff member, Bob, when a customer's ball successfully entered a fish bowl–at which time the staff member then transferred the fish into a sealed plastic container for the customer. In order to help Ed to remember his responsibilities, a sign indicating (a) the number of correct tickets to collect and (b) the number of correct balls to disburse was placed in Ed's visual field behind the booth's counter. Additionally, since Ed experienced occasional balance problems while leaning forward, he was provided with a long-arm reaching device having wide suction grips in order to retrieve ping-pong balls from the ground without having to bend. These adaptations successfully allowed Ed to operate the booth with relatively little assistance from his surrogate big-brother.

SAL: MIXED MESSAGES FROM THE REHAB TEAM. THE REBUILDING OF ADULT MALE GENDER ROLES (TIER 1)

Perhaps out of all of the four men, Sal had experienced the most extensive disruption in his post-injury male role participation. The loss of such roles as son, brother, husband, worker, friend, and independent home maintainer–and the loss of the relationships and activities that supported those roles–was a traumatic experience for Sal.

> It was like being plucked from my life and plopped down someplace I didn't want to be. And everything I knew to be mine was no longer a part of my life.

After injury the attempts that Sal made to rebuild several of his lost roles were unsuccessful. Of particular concern to him was his inability to obtain independent apartment living and resume dating relationships. When the intervention began, Sal expressed considerable dissatisfaction with his rehabilitation placement and frequently verbalized a desire to leave.

> They [Sal's TBI treatment team members] set me up. They send me to the apartments; then they send me back. They discouraged my dating several of the women here. I don't feel like they're helping me to be independent and I don't feel like I'm being rehabilitated.

Sal's relationship with his brother and mother were severely strained. While he had not spoken with his brother in the last five years, Sal did report that he managed to maintain a relationship with his mother, despite feelings of betrayal. Sal expressed that his relationship with his mother was unsatisfactory and often hurtful. Nevertheless, he often initiated phone contact with his mother and requested to be taken to her home for weekend visits–a request that his mother rarely indulged. When asked why Sal continued to seek frequent contact with his mother despite his feelings of resentment and hurt, Sal replied, "She's the only family I have left. I have no one else really. So I'm willing to put up with her abuse I guess because I have no one else."

Sal reported that he had no friends at the TBI rehabilitation facility, stating that he shared nothing in common with his housemates other than the head injury–a similarity that he preferred to forget. The portrait that Sal painted of himself was that of a man very much alone, disconnected from friends, family members, and the larger society in which his role as an independent man was no longer certain.

Ironically, Sal's friendship was readily sought by other male clients who respected both Sal's wisdom and life experience. However, Sal expressed that he was unable to find individuals residing at the facility who could match his cognitive communication skills and thus provide an appropriate level of intellectual stimulation. Although Sal's friendship was desired at the rehabilitation facility, he nevertheless felt alone and lacking any opportunity to rebuild the relationships that could support his roles as an adult man.

One of the first relationships that Sal attempted to develop through his participation in the intervention was a mentor-protégé relationship with the facility's neuropsychologist, Dr. Murphy. Because Sal had not possessed a strong relationship with an older male since the death of his father–which occurred shortly after his first TBI–we believed that Sal would benefit from the opportunity to build a relationship with a male mentor who could act as both a guide and a friend. Initially, Sal and Dr. Murphy met twice weekly for lunch in community restaurants–as it was important for Sal to develop relationships in which he could step outside of his role as a client in a TBI rehabilitation center.

> Dr. Murphy is like a friend to me. He treats me with respect, like I'm a grown man and he doesn't talk down to me like the other staff people. I don't feel like I'm just a client with him. He respects my experience and that I had a life before this head injury. And I respect him for that because with him I feel like a whole man, not some freak.

Sal's Denial and Externalization of Responsibility

While Sal had grown to accept his mentor's extension of friendship, he had not as readily responded to the overtures of other males residing at the facility who also sought Sal's companionship. Sal's unwillingness to pursue friendships with other male clients may have been related to his discomfort with his own TBI. The cognitive deficits and physical limitations exhibited more overtly by other clients may have been difficult for Sal to accept in himself. Despite the existence of documented cognitive difficulties–difficulties that contributed to the apartment fire that precipitated Sal's return to the group home–Sal continued to deny that he possessed any deficit areas. At the same time, he eschewed contact with the friends he had made while living in the apartment program, convinced that his friends now judged him to be inferior as a result of his perceived lowered status as a group home resident. At the outset of the intervention, it appeared that Sal's perception of himself as an adult man had become further damaged as a result of his inability to maintain apartment living. Not having the skills to understand his emotions–a skill deficit that was likely compounded by his neurologic injury–Sal displaced his anger onto staff members and therapists whom he blamed for his recent setbacks.

The Making of a Mentor: Rebuilding Self-Respect

It appeared that Sal would benefit from the opportunity to assume a surrogate big-brother role with younger male clients who could express an appreciation for and validate the high level social skills that Sal did possess. However, when I approached Sal regarding the possibility of assisting other male residents, Sal expressed that he had nothing of worth to contribute to others. Sal agreed instead to accompany me while I participated in social activities with several other males residing in both the campus units and the group homes. On these occasions, Sal held doors open, assisted with menu reading and ordering, and answered a myriad of questions ranging from dating and women to old rock music bands. To the younger male clients, Sal was a sophisticated older brother figure who possessed world experience. While Sal was uncertain of his standing among his pre-injury relationships and roles, he was beginning to build an identity as a role model within the TBI facility.

> Since my accident I never really thought of myself as a role model, after all I **need** [his emphasis] help–isn't that why I'm here [spoken with sarcasm]? People always looked up to me before [my TBI], but not now. But, if I can help someone then I want to be able to. That's really the only thing that makes me feel good.

The ability to help others encouraged Sal to reassess personal competencies that he had formerly devalued. Once again in his life, Sal began to internalize the respect that others–including both his mentor and younger male friends–now demonstrated toward him.

> I feel like I did before my first accident when I felt competent being a provider for my family. I used to think that taking care of others meant providing for them financially. Really though, now I see that you can take care of people in different ways; I mean

not just with money. I mean, I appreciate my ability to help other people, but now I help them differently–like helping [client's name] to get outside; if no staff is around I'll help out. It makes me feel good. . . . The only thing that I can compare it to in my life before my accident was how my father treated me. He was always there as a friend to me; not just to me but to everyone he dealt with. He was a good man. And I'd like to be a friend now to [client's name] like that too. I'd like to be the kind of man like my father was.

While Sal had established a surrogate big-brother role with several of the younger male clients who sought his fellowship, he had not as yet begun to develop reciprocal peer relationships in which he too could benefit from others' care and nurturance. Even Sal's volunteer position at a neighborhood nursing home–in which he served as a client transport–further supported his identity as a caregiver and provider. It appeared that Sal was most comfortable in roles in which he offered care rather than received it–a personality characteristic that was congruent with Sal's reported pre-injury roles. For Sal, the ability to accept assistance concomitantly required the admittance of vulnerability–an emotion that he may have been unprepared or unwilling to confront in himself presently. Human beings are not solitary creatures, however, and Sal's insistence that he needed no one appeared protective and limiting.

The Courtship of Sal and Ann

I believed that Sal would benefit from developing friendships with other male clients with whom he shared similar life experiences and present functional abilities. Sal, however, was adamant that he neither desired to reacquaint himself with his former friends at the apartment program nor develop friendships with the men living in his group home whom he considered to be less cognitively competent. Conversely, Sal was not hesitant to accept an introduction to a female client, and I readily utilized this opportunity to acquaint Sal with a woman who resided in a community group home located one block from Sal's residence. Coincidentally, this particular female client, Ann, was Sal's age and sustained her injury in the same year as Sal. While she relied upon a wheelchair and electronic mobile scooter for ambulation, she had also achieved independent community travel status and could easily access local restaurants, shopping centers, and movie theaters. Sal and Ann began dating steadily, spending all of their free time together as couples often do in the early stages of relationships.

While Sal was now receiving the care and nurturance that we had hoped for him, he continued to lack reciprocal peer relationships with other males through which he could assume a role as a friend. I worried–much in a parental-like way–that Sal had become dependent upon Ann for most of his emotional support and companionship. I was also concerned that Sal would be left without an emotional support system if his relationship with Ann deteriorated. Not wanting to create a failure experience for Sal, I pressed him further to develop friendships with other male clients who could become a part of his supportive network.

Expanding the Supportive Network

While Sal continued to remain disinterested in spending time with other male clients–especially if it decreased his contact with Ann–he was more agreeable to the idea of inviting other clients to join him and Ann for dinner. In this way Sal was able to increase his exposure to other clients in an attempt to build friendships. Apparently, familiarity breeds liking; several of Ann's male friends–for whom Sal initially expressed dislike–began to regularly join Ann and Sal for dinner in local community restaurants. Sal even began to independently seek the company of these men when Ann was working or unavailable for other reasons. Additionally, Sal reported that he no longer felt the need to call his mother weekly nor request to visit at her home.

> My socialization is much more personally satisfying now since I've been seeing Ann and becoming friends with [several male clients]. Mother's negative actions and words don't seem to bother me as much; well, I'm not really having as much contact with her as I used to. . . . I guess I don't feel that I need her so much; I mean I don't feel as much by myself as I did. . . . I've learned there are people in this world who can be trusted, I think. I don't have to keep knocking my head against a wall trying to have a relationship with Mother if it isn't gonna be there. And God knows my brains have been knocked around enough anyway.

During the four months of intervention, Sal and Ann's relationship became increasingly inseparable. Although Sal had built friendships with two other male clients and had developed a caring relationship with his mentor, I continued to wonder what would happen to Sal if his relationship with Ann began to falter. All relationships are subject to the stresses of ordinary life events and Sal and Ann's relationship was no exception. In the third month of the study, Ann was notified by her treatment team members that she had gained sufficient independence in her daily living skills and would be transferred to a shared community apartment upon the next available occupancy. While Ann was thrilled at the prospect of attaining a role as an independent home maintainer in the community, Sal appeared uncomfortable with Ann's possible change in status and began again to verbalize his desire to leave the facility.

In the cultural system in which Sal was raised, he was likely socialized to believe that as a man, he would naturally assume the roles of an independent home maintainer–a role that encompassed financial provision for both a wife and family. Ann's ability to attain a role that Sal had recently lost was probably perceived by Sal as a threat to his adult male role status. Through discussion of his concerns with his mentor and I, Sal revealed his fear that Ann, once having moved to the apartments, would look down upon him and end their relationship: "Why would she [Ann] want to date a man beneath her? She'll probably meet someone in the apartments and I'll be outa the picture." More often, Sal displaced his feelings of inferiority onto his treatment team members whom he blamed for his inability to maintain apartment living.

> If things don't change I'm gonna leave. They [treatment team members] don't know what they're doing. I should be in the apartments, not in a group home. I'm not being rehabilitated here. I'm gonna leave and take Ann with me.

Ann's move to the apartment program was not imminent and would be unlikely to occur for another year. As the frenzy concerning Ann's possible move diminished and Sal's fears began to recede, Sal became more receptive to my attempts to help him to re-establish adult male roles. Perhaps the perceived threat of losing Ann encouraged Sal to understand the importance of building a supportive network of several others, rather than relying upon one person for emotional sustenance. In the last month of the intervention, staff members reported that Sal more commonly sought his male friends for social activities outside of his relationship with Ann. Sal also spent more time at the main facility campus to provide assistance to several of the younger clients with whom he had formed a surrogate big-brother relationship. It appeared that Sal was learning the skills necessary to balance a dating/courtship role with a variety of friendship and extended-family roles.

The Master Craftsman Returns

As mentioned previously, Sal was fortunate to have re-obtained a community member role as a volunteer in a local nursing home–a role that was both personally meaningful and provided the opportunity for Sal to use his skills to assist others. However, while Sal had assumed a big-brother surrogate role with several male clients who resided on the main facility campus, he did not possess any formal adult roles within the TBI facility through which he could receive recognition as a competent adult man. Sal, who had indulged pre-injury talents as a carpenter and craftsman, expressed interest in helping the recreational therapist during the bi-weekly arts and crafts night at the main facility campus. In this role, Sal distributed supplies and assisted clients having cognitive and physical limitations to create handicrafts from a variety of materials. Once again, Sal's contribution was greatly valued by the clients residing on the main facility campus, many of whom respected Sal's apparent sophistication, life experience, and social interaction skills. On the evenings that Sal did not attend, the recreational therapist reported that clients who normally displayed interest in the crafts group did not wish to participate. When Sal was made aware of his popularity and respect, he appeared surprised and uncomfortable.

> I didn't realize that anyone cared if I showed up or not [to the crafts group]. I figured I was just another pair of hands. But I guess I have to admit it makes me feel pretty good.

The recognition and respect that Sal attained through his role in the crafts group further helped him to reshape his identity as an adult man.

> I definitely feel like I have more responsibilities now than at any other time since my accident. And yeah, that's a pretty good feeling. But I would imagine it would make anybody feel good to have a life where they were doing things, meaningful things; not just sitting around killing time. At least I'd rather be active and have adult responsibilities. I liked my life when I was independent and took care of my responsibilities myself. My volunteer jobs in

[the nursing home] and here [in the crafts group], I guess, let me be responsible for others. And helping others really is the only time when I feel completely separate from being a client, like I'm not a client anymore; it's like I'm a man like any other man.

A Contract for the Return to Apartment Living

While Sal reported greater comfort with his identity as an adult man as a result of assuming new roles, his status as a community group home resident continued to cause him considerable distress. For Sal, an adult male status would not be complete without obtaining independent community living. Sal's rehabilitation treatment team members, however, were adamantly convinced that Sal's safety issues and tendency to resume drug use caused him to be a poor candidate for independent apartment living. Ironically, while Sal's treatment team members were able to identify the deficits that impeded his independence, Sal was not receiving appropriate intervention to remediate his deficit areas. I suggested that Sal receive some type of drug abuse intervention and regularly attend AA or MICA (Mentally Ill Chemical Abusers) support group meetings. Additionally, since Sal did not wish to stop smoking cigarettes, I suggested that the apartment program become smoke-free–as both the community group homes and main facility campus units had become (i.e., clients are required to smoke outside and place cigarette butts in appropriate outdoor containers provided by the facility). I further recommended that Sal and his treatment team members create a contractual agreement stating that Sal's ability to re-obtain–and maintain–apartment living would be contingent upon adherence to two specific criteria: (a) attendance at a drug abuse/support group and (b) agreement to smoke outside of the apartment building. As the intervention came to an end, Sal's treatment team members were considering the idea of a contract supporting Sal's return to the apartment program, but no decisions had been finalized.

SAL: "TO CONNECT TO OTHERS MEANS EMOTIONAL PAIN." THE PARTICIPATION IN ACTIVITIES THAT SUPPORTED THE ACQUISITION OF MALE GENDER ROLES (TIER 2)

Unlike the other men, Sal did not possess restrictions concerning phone usage, community travel, and money management. In fact, Sal was one of the few clients in the TBI community group home program who possessed his own phone line and managed a savings and checking account with minimal assistance from a private accountant. Additionally, unlike the other three men, Sal demonstrated high level social interaction skills, including the ability to independently extend social invitations and arrange social gatherings. At the beginning of the intervention, however, Sal was not using his social skills to build relationships with others, but rather spent most of his free time alone. The activities that Sal used to meet others–dining out alone and initiating conversations with restaurant employees–did not truly provide the opportunity for him to build meaningful relationships. In hindsight, it was apparent that Sal may not have wished to build relationships deeper than acquaintances, as all of Sal's close bonds both pre- and post-injury were largely characterized by pain and betrayal. Sal may have decided that superficial acquaintances were less hurtful than deeper ties, and thus chose to limit his emotional closeness to others. It was discouraging to observe Sal restrict his contact with others when he in fact possessed the skills to build a network of friends and extended family.

Allowing a Mentor to Get Close

Sal's relationship with his mentor was the first bond that he allowed to develop since he had moved back from the apartment program. As mentioned, it was important for his mentor to provide the opportunity for Sal to participate in activities that were separate from the TBI facility and Sal's role as a client. Activities that Sal and his mentor shared included eating in community restaurants, attending home and building conventions, and shopping in community malls. These activities provided an avenue for Sal to enact his role as an adult man. Shopping for clothes, cologne, and other men's grooming products was an activity that Sal particularly enjoyed as he was fastidious about his appearance and often expressed concern that he had lost his masculine physique.

> I like shopping for clothes with [the author] because she can give me a woman's opinion like when I used to go shopping with my wives. They'd tell me what looks good and what doesn't. . . . How I look is really important to me. It always has been ever since the polio. When I was in my early 20s I was pretty muscu-

lar and big. Ever since my accident it hasn't been that way. First I gained a lot of weight–I mean **a lot** [his emphasis] of weight. And ever since then I've been really conscious of how I look. Now they [treatment team members] say I'm too thin. I'm 6'2" and 180 pounds. I miss my muscles but I'm in a lot of pain most of the time and can't lift major weights like I used to. And the stretching exercises I do for my back don't really add muscle bulk–not like I used to have. And on top of all that I'm going gray [laughs]. But you'd never know it cause I color the gray out.

Budgeting for a New Lifestyle

While Sal managed his own finances with the assistance of a private accountant, he did not appear to utilize any particular budgetary system to organize his weekly expenses. As Sal began to increase his spending in the community as a result of greater participation in activities with his mentor and Ann, the need to help Sal budget his funds became more apparent. Sal was receiving a combined monthly sum of $450.00 from his social security income and an insurance settlement annuity. His financial strategy was to spend the monthly allowance until it was depleted–at which time Sal either ate in the community group home or, more commonly, skipped meals. Sal and I began to use a budget planning book to organize Sal's monthly and weekly expenses. At the beginning of each week, Sal would estimate his financial expenses and withdraw only that amount from his account. If he found that his expenses exceeded his initial estimate, Sal would then withdraw a greater cash amount, careful not to exceed his weekly limit of $112.00. In this way, Sal learned how to budget his finances to maintain consistent participation in the activities that supported his adult male roles.

I don't know what I was thinking before [using a financial budget]. I guess after the accident my motto was spend it while you got it. And at the end of the month when my money ran out I figured I enjoyed it while I had it. But this [planning to have money throughout the entire month] is a lot better. Especially because now I'm planning someone else's [Ann's] social activities too and if I run out of money because I didn't plan ahead we won't be able to do things we both enjoy doing.

Getting Organized

Despite Sal's short-term memory deficits he had proficiently learned to use a memory/date book to record appointments and important events. The ability to schedule and carryout planned activities significantly helped Sal to rebuild a repertoire of activities through which he could express his male gender identity. However, while Sal's weekly schedule book was neatly organized, he did not concomitantly maintain a usable phone and address book. Consequently, in the early days of his relationship with Ann, Sal often missed appointments with Ann because he had misplaced her phone number and address. Similarly, when Sal began to develop a surrogate big-brother role with several younger male clients residing on the main facility campus, he frequently was unable to carry through with promises to call them, as he had recorded their phone numbers in a phone book that lacked any system of categorization. For example, Sal recorded entries according to an individual's last or first name–but with no consistent pattern. When a page became full with addresses, he then recorded new entries in the margins and page corners–a strategy that further exacerbated Sal's poor visual scanning skills. Sal's phone book listed the names of individuals whom he had met in the course of his rehabilitation but now no longer remembered. However, while Sal's phone book was unusable for present purposes, the large array of phone numbers and addresses that he had collected over the years attested to his sociable nature and ability to develop friendships.

Sal and I organized a new phone and address book in accordance with a specific categorization system that was printed in bold letters in the book's front and back covers. If Sal knew an individual by his or her first name he would record that person's phone number by first name only to enhance his recall. Conversely, if Sal referred to an individual by a surname (as in Dr. Murphy), he recorded that person's entry by his or her last name. Names were now recorded only in available lined spaces and not in page margins or corners. Additionally, names of individuals with whom Sal was no longer in contact were weeded out while commonly used phone numbers were highlighted in yellow. Entries also included a description of Sal's relationship to the individual to enhance his recall. A page of names and phone numbers of Sal's treatment team members was created. So too was a page listing the phone numbers of each main facility campus unit and community group home residence. These adaptations enabled Sal to use his phone book to maintain a network of supportive relationships through which to express his masculine identity.

> I always had a lot of friends before my head injury. It was just who I was. I feel more like the guy I used to be, now, being able to have friends again, or I guess even wanting to be around people again.

Preparing to Be Sexual Partners: Sal and Ann

Sal also expressed concern regarding the development of a sexual relationship with Ann. While Ann and Sal felt comfortable with the privacy afforded by Ann's community group home, Sal's back pain and Ann's physical limitations posed difficulties for the couple's engagement in sexual activity. A member of the nursing staff and I discussed positions for optimal comfort and reduced pain with both Ann and Sal. Because of Ann's physical limitations, she could not maintain an unsupported sitting position, thus requiring her to assume either a sidelying or supine position (on her back) during sexual activity. Sal, however, could neither maintain a prone position (on stomach) supported on his arms nor a supine position due to severe back pain. Consequently, one position that accommodated each was a sidelying position supported laterally by pillows.

Additionally, energy conservation techniques were discussed with Ann and Sal including consideration of the effects of medication and fatigue level upon the planning of sexual activity. Safe sex practices were reviewed at this time as well. This information helped Sal and Ann to participate in the activities of an adult sexual relationship–a privilege of adulthood that is often elusive for individuals residing in supportive living facilities.

> Some of the planning sort of, how can I say, decreases the spontaneity, although at my age spontaneity isn't always there anyway. It's not like when I was 20. But it's still gratifying. I'm glad we can have this part of our relationship together . . . . It makes me feel more normal, like the person I used to be. And I want Ann to get a chance to see the real me, not just the head injured part of me.

Chapter 6

Greater Satisfaction
with Post-Injury Male Gender Roles:
The Men's Self-Reports

After their four-month intervention, each of the men were interviewed to determine if they were more satisfied with their male gender roles. Common themes emerged throughout the men's separate interviews: (a) greater satisfaction with post-injury male gender roles, (b) attaining personal goals, (c) feeling more like a member of society, (d) feeling like oneself again, (e) learning about oneself as an adult man, (f) greater comfort with the use of help-seeking behaviors, (g) contributing to others through community member and extended-family roles, (h) fear of staff reprisal, and (i) unfulfilled expectations. These themes are discussed below using the men's own words to illustrate their shared sentiments.

GREATER SATISFACTION WITH POST-INJURY MALE
GENDER ROLES: BEING A MAN AGAIN

One theme that consistently emerged in the men's post-intervention interviews was their greater satisfaction with newly rebuilt post-injury male gender roles. Prior to the intervention, each of the men reported that being a client had become their primary role–a role so consuming

[Haworth co-indexing entry note]: "Greater Satisfaction with Post-Injury Male Gender Roles: The Men's Self-Reports." Gutman, Sharon A. Co-published simultaneously in *Occupational Therapy in Mental Health* (The Haworth Press, Inc.) Vol. 15, No. 3/4, 2000, pp. 111-126; and: *Brain Injury and Gender Role Strain: Rebuilding Adult Lifestyles After Injury* (Sharon A. Gutman) The Haworth Press, Inc., 2000, pp. 111-126. Single or multiple copies of this article are available for a fee from The Haworth Document Delivery Service [1-800-342-9678, 9:00 a.m. - 5:00 p.m. (EST). E-mail address: getinfo@haworth pressinc.com].

111

that Rudy compared it to a professional career. After the intervention, the men reported deriving greater satisfaction from having successfully rebuilt several social roles that were lost post-injury (e.g., friend, community member, extended-family member). In particular, the men expressed that having the opportunity to participate in roles other than that of a client enabled them to feel more like adult men.

It's really been important to me to have roles other than just being a client. Being able to go out to dinner with Ann or my role as a client transport at the nursing home. These things have made me feel better about the way I feel about my life now. It feels more like an adult man's [life]. (Sal)

Me [and two other male clients] were just sitting around and bullshitting. It was nice camaraderie–like three friends who really care about each other. It was a man thing, you know? Just hanging out with the guys. Not doing anything really, just shooting the breeze, hanging out with friends. You don't know how good that is for me–to have that [role] back in my life, being like a man's man. I wanted that for a long time. (Rudy)

I think [the role of] being a brother is a lot more satisfying to me now, maybe than it ever was, or at least since I can remember. I feel accepted as a brother now. I feel like, yeah I *am* [his emphasis] a brother. That feels really good. (Jay)

Being able to walk around the community, meet my friends at restaurants, call my friends up [on the phone] makes me feel like an independent adult man. I've wanted to be an independent man. I'm 30 years old. It's about time. (Ed)

Just to be able to sit with a lady over a nice dinner–even if she's just a friend, I don't care. It's such a difference [from when Rudy was prevented from having contact with women]. It makes all the difference in the world–you don't know. I feel like a human being again. (Rudy)

ATTAINING PERSONAL GOALS: SOCIAL HOPES FULFILLED

The men also expressed that through the rebuilding of male gender roles and activities, they had attained several personal goals for which they had given up hope post-injury. Such personal goals included developing a dating relationship, building friendships, and participating in meaningful work.

> Well, I wanted to date again [after his TBI] but I never seemed to have luck with women after my first wife. It was like she [first wife] cursed me with women forever. I just figured this is the way it's gonna be. . . . I guess I'm lucky to have met Ann. I didn't think it [developing a dating relationship] would happen again, but I'm glad it did. (Sal)

> Lyn taught me how to be friends with girls–how to act with women. I'm more comfortable now with talking to women. I'm shy; it used to be hard for me to talk to women. Just to come up with something to say or look them in the eye. Now I can hold a conversation with a woman. I talk to Arlene every week. It makes me feel good. I always wanted to be able to talk more easy with women like the other guys. (Ed)

> I've grown less shy. I get along more with people. I'm more friendly with people at work. I wanted to have friends. I used to not talk to nobody. I learned to speak up more, to be assertive. (Ed)

For Rudy, the attainment of male friendships was bittersweet. While Rudy was able to rebuild the male friendships that had not been a part of his life since his accident, he also lost the closest male friend he had ever known throughout his life–his father. One week after the intervention period ended, Rudy's father died suddenly from complications resulting from a chronic heart condition.

> I been wanting to have buddies for a long time. And boy, thank God I got em now cause the camaraderie and support from my friends has made it [the death of his father] more bearable.

Similarly, Jay expressed satisfaction with his ability to participate in creative writing again–a long desired goal. Toward the end of the intervention period, Jay's mother had shown a sample of his writing to a professional writer who expressed interest in assisting Jay to compile a book of personal thoughts about his experience of head injury. By the end of the intervention Jay had successfully rebuilt meaningful work into his post-injury life and was now embarking upon a new creative endeavor–writing a book–that he had only recently believed to be an impossibility.

> I was in a rut. I didn't see how I could fulfill my dreams. Writing seemed like, it seemed like I would never write again. So many things we combat with diligence and we're grateful that we took the pain and frustration cause it pays off in the end. At least it's paid off for me. I'm fulfilling my expectations pretty much now. I'm feeding myself with fulfillment with goals I had for myself. These things are the dessert of my life. I didn't expect them but they've made me feel better about my life. It's like a present, something to look forward to. It's one of the rewards of life from working hard and these are the treats.

Several of the men also indicated that meeting personal goals enabled them to feel a greater sense of competency. Moreover, the opportunity for family members to observe the men in male adult roles was reported to be highly meaningful. The participants expressed that they felt less of a burden on family members and appreciated the opportunity for family members to acknowledge the men's greater skill proficiency.

> Having more friends, writing again–this brings out a feeling of competence. I want my family to see the productive side of me, that I can be more independent and not burden my parents as much. I think my mom was surprised but also proud to see me be writing again. (Jay)

> I can take care of myself. Now I can show my parents that I'm an adult man. I have friends and a girlfriend. I work. I can take my own money and go out to eat with friends. (Ed)

For Rudy, the opportunity to demonstrate his participation in newly rebuilt male roles before his father's death, carried considerable personal importance and helped him to resolve concerns he had expressed regarding burdening his father.

> I think that my dad really felt and thought of me in the realm of, "My son Rudy, he's at a more advanced, okay place in his reha-

bilitation." It was one of those father-son things, that he perceived me as coming along more towards the end [of his father's life]. I felt better about how he was starting to feel better about me, his son, that he didn't have to worry so much what would happen to me. I felt he had more trust and confidence in me, in my ability to take care of myself and have the kinda lifestyle that reflects the man I am. And that really makes me tear up–you only have one dad, you know what I'm saying? I don't know how long it took me to get over my mom's death a while back, but I feel a lot better that my dad saw me at this stage in my rehab before he died. I wish my mom had too. That really hurts, cause my rehab, well it was for me, but it was as much for my dad also because he was always so interested in my rehab. It meant so much to him.

FEELING MORE LIKE A MEMBER OF SOCIETY: "LIKE A NORMAL CITIZEN"

Along with meeting personal goals, the participants also reported that they felt more like members of society. Spending greater amounts of time within the community, engaged in socially accepted adult roles and activities enabled the men to feel a greater part of society in ways they were unable to within the group home setting.

It's made such a difference, being able to go up town [in the community], up to the shopping center, have dinner with friends . . . . Here's my rehab [draws an invisible line with his hands], and here's the end of rehab. I'm just about at a point where I feel like I'm stepping into being a societal member again. (Rudy)

In addition to feeling more like members of society, the men expressed that a greater sense of normalcy had re-entered their lives.

It's nice to be out in public, doing things like a normal citizen. Doing things it takes to live like a normal person–normal things which seem small, but which are very big and basic parts of life in our society. Like maybe meeting friends for a meal or seeing a movie together. (Jay)

How I feel now, this is as close to normal as I've felt since my head injury. (Sal)

Being here [at the rehabilitation facility] is like a counterfeit lifestyle, an artificial one I mean. It's clinicized, it's an unnatural lifestyle. Because you don't have a normal lifestyle or any choice in what you do with your time. You're always here or there because it's your therapy or you have an appointment with this person or that person. You never get to make a decision about how to spend your time–what activities to do. But now that's changed to some degree. I can't even express to you what a change in lifestyle this is, having some ability to see friends or take a lady out to dinner. It's normal, like any other person in society. (Rudy)

FEELING LIKE ONESELF AGAIN:
REBUILDING A PERSONALIZED LIFESTYLE

The men also reported that they had begun to feel like themselves again; that is, they felt a greater congruency between their internal perceptions of themselves and their external post-injury roles.

When I first had my head injury I felt like I had been taken out of my life and put into another person's life. I'm finally getting back some of me, doing things I thought I'd be doing as an adult man. (Sal)

Writing and having friends has been for me, well it's let me feel more like how I am naturally, my own nature I mean. I feel like who I think I really am or could be if given the chance. (Jay)

Rudy, too, expressed the idea that he was beginning to rebuild a lifestyle that more closely matched his internal perception of his ideal self. For Rudy, it was doubly important that his father had the opportunity to witness this ideal self before his father's death.

I've been married to this head injury for the last twenty-some years. I'm just starting to get back a little bit of who I really feel I am. And I felt my dad got a chance to glimpse the real me before his death–I mean, to see me more like the man I feel myself to be. And my dad knew me inside out. I think he got a chance to say, "Yeah, that's my son Rudy, the man I knew he could be."

LEARNING ABOUT ONESELF AS AN ADULT MAN: THE EMERGENCE OF AN ADULT SELF

In addition to feeling a greater congruency between their internal perceptions of themselves and their post-injury roles, the men reported that they had begun to learn more about themselves through their newly rebuilt roles and activities. For these men, the occurrence of a TBI during the ages of 18-30 disrupted the developmental transition from adolescent to adult roles. Consequently, the men did not possess the roles through which they could know themselves as adult men. The opportunity to rebuild adult male gender roles and activities enabled the men to learn more about their adult proclivities, preferences and dislikes, and values.

> I like people. I like having friends. I never really knew that about myself. I always thought I was a loner. Cause it was hard to make friends. Now I have more friends and I like it. I like having friends instead of being alone all the time. (Ed)

> You know I always had an inkling that this was me–that I was different from how my life looked to people on the outside. I'm a 48 year old man and I'm just beginning to find out who I really am. Well, I guess better late than never. I have a greater understanding and perception of myself and who I really am through these roles. Take for example painting and ceramics. I never knew I was an artist. Painting is an avenue of my Italian-American artistry. It makes me feel like a man–like Picasso, a man full of passion to express. It's one of the most fulfilling [roles] I have now. (Rudy)

> Writing has helped me to get to know myself better. It's changed the way I see myself as intelligent, curious, interested, and motivated to improve myself and make the most of my personal assets. I have greater self-confidence now. I'm learning about myself. I'm discovering new territory in my imagination. I like the idea of knowing there are things in me that no one expected–and that I didn't even expect. I've discovered more of myself and there's a lot more that can be developed. And there are a lot of ways to discover it, I learned. It's given me hope that I can reach some of my dreams. (Jay)

Moreover, several of the men indicated that they had begun to rethink their definitions of what it means to be a man. Sal, very articulately, attempted to describe the change process that transpired as he reconsidered and altered his views about being an adult man.

> Years ago my role as a husband was to make money for her [his first wife] to spend. At the time, I enjoyed providing for her because I didn't realize how many more roles could be rewarding to me, as maybe I see better now. After my injury I tried real hard to be the kind of man I was before my accident–and I screwed up, I made mistakes like anybody I think. How much money I made, how many homes I owned–that's what was most important to me [before injury]. Now, giving to others is very important to me. Helping others as I was helped when I needed it. And doing something with my time that I enjoy and makes me feel good about myself. I don't need to earn a lot of money to feel like a man–don't get me wrong, it would be nice. But it doesn't mean the same thing anymore. I'd much rather spend my time volunteering to help the clients at [the main facility campus] or the seniors at the nursing home.

Ed also expressed that he had begun to reconsider his definition of male adulthood. When Ed first began his participation in the intervention, he believed that he could only achieve happiness by attaining the adult male roles of husband and father. At the end of the intervention period, Ed was able to consider alternative ways in which he could create fulfilling roles as an adult man.

> I used to think if only I could be married, I'd be happy. I'd still like to get married but I can be happy even if I don't get married, too. It won't be the end of the world if I don't get married. As long as I have my friends and my family I'll be happy. They love me. I don't feel alone like I used to.

GREATER COMFORT WITH HELP-SEEKING BEHAVIORS: "IT'S OKAY TO ADMIT YOU NEED HELP"

One of the most dramatic changes that occurred during the intervention concerned the men's greater comfort with the use of help-seeking behaviors. Characteristic of many males with head injury the men reported that prior to the intervention they did not consistently seek staff or peer assistance when problems occurred. Consequently, the men felt alone in their experience of head injury and failed to utilize appropriate resources to solve problems. The failure to utilize others for assistance with problem-solving may have been related to pre-injury socialized behavioral patterns–as it is common for males in western society to refrain from using help-seeking behaviors and to isolate themselves in times of crisis (Bem, 1993; Lindsey, 1994).

In the intervention, the opportunity to develop both friendships with fellow clients and relationships with male mentors provided the men with appropriate sources from whom to seek advice and support.

> I feel comfortable talking to Bob [mentor/surrogate big-brother] about my problems. He's always willing to listen and help. I feel lucky to be able to go to him for help. (Ed)

> I don't always open up with others, I mean about my feelings and problems. That's the way I am. I used to be fully open with everyone and I saw how they took advantage of me. I got hurt emotionally as well as financially. So it's not easy for me to open up or ask someone else for help. But Dr. Murphy [mentor] is like an instructor to me. Many times, many different suggestions that he's made assisted me in making my own decisions. He's been a real guide to me and I trust him. (Sal)

> I appreciate my friendships with [several male clients] because I look to them for different answers if I have a problem. I depend on their past experience, especially if it's experience that I don't have. And I ask them their advice and then compare it to my situation. . . . I'm more willing now to ask for their advice because I think I've become more cautious about who to ask. And I think I've found some people I can trust. (Sal)

> The support I got from Eric [mentor] and several [male clients] has made a big difference in helping me adjust and get through this hard time what with the loss of my dad. It's really made me count my blessings for having these guys around. (Rudy)

Three sub-themes emerged as a result of the men's greater comfort with the use of help-seeking behaviors: (a) feeling a sense of shared experience and affinity, (b) feeling understood and accepted, and (c) filling a void. The men indicated that by seeking help from appropriate sources they found others with whom they experienced a sense of kinship and personal affirmation.

Camaraderie: Feeling a Sense of Shared Experience and Affinity

Seeking social support enabled the men to observe that others shared their experience and concerns. The idea that individuals can feel a sense of affinity with others experiencing similar situations was first considered by Yalom (1970), who noted that a therapeutic group process could provide members with a feeling of universality–that is, a feeling that one's concerns are not unique but rather shared by others. Barrett (1978) found that universality could be facilitated outside of a group setting by having one other person with whom to share similar experiences; and in fact, most of the men's experiences of universality occurring during the intervention period emerged in one-to-one relationships with mentors or friends.

> I've really gotten significantly tight and close with [male client's name]. And it's always nice to have someone going through the same thing as whatever you're going through. You're able to give your perception and compare it to his and you know, come up with a different perspective, a different way of looking at things. Having someone I can feel like-minded with is, well [male client's] life experience is comparative to mine–we're cut from the same mold. It's a gift from God to be able to find someone who knows what I'm going through. It just makes me feel like not such a doofus to know that somebody I respect has gone through the same thing. (Rudy)

Feeling Understood and Accepted as a Friend

Likewise, having at least one other person with whom to discuss concerns enabled the men to feel understood and accepted–a significant occurrence, as most of the men initially reported feeling alone in their experience of head injury, misunderstood by others in their immediate environment, and alienated from the larger society.

> I used to feel like everyone hated me before [the intervention period]. Now I have friends. I feel better about myself. I feel that others feel better about me and want to be around me. (Ed)

> Ann is a good friend that I'm able to be myself with. We're both disabled, we have this in common. We're two disabled people that

society looks upon and points a finger at. So in that respect she knows what it's like to be head injured. I enjoy her company and I feel like she knows me well and accepts me for who I am. (Sal)

Jay, who at the start of the intervention indicated that he was uncertain if his friends were real or "sympathy friends," now felt more assured that his friendship was indeed valued by others.

Friendships are a needed psychological experience. It makes me feel good [having friends]. It's given me peace of mind. I feel accepted for who I am and kinda appreciated by others as an okay kinda guy.

Interestingly Rudy, whose comments were often couched in war terminology attributed his greater feeling of acceptance to having an "ally" upon whom to rely.

He's [male client] a man about my age and he has the same experience and such and desires and thoughts about life similar to myself. And that hits me where I live. He's someone I can relate to, being in the same position I'm in. He's like an ally. And he takes the edge off things for me. You know, like if something happens, if I did something that I goofed up, he makes me feel less stupid. And also if I did something good, he's there to give me the pat on the back I don't give myself.

The acceptance that Sal found in his role as an extended-family big brother helped him to replace his desire to seek acceptance among his peers at a local bar.

Before my accident–and also after my accident too–I would go to the bar and everyone there would know me as a friend. It was part of my social activity. It's sort of like that now on campus [the rehabilitation facility]. The younger guys know me and ask me to come by. And actually, that's not such a bad feeling [feeling accepted by clients with TBI].

Caring Mentors Fill a Void

Several of the clients also indicated that having someone from whom to seek advice, filled a void that had been created long ago, sometimes prior to injury.

I never really had a real father or brother, you know, someone I could sort of turn to for male advice. It's nice now to have someone to fill that need. Even if I don't see him as much as I'd like to. (Jay)

For Rudy and Sal, the post-injury loss of prominent male figures in their lives created a void that was, in part, filled by the development of a relationship with a male mentor who was familiar with the head injury experience.

When I'm in a situation and such I go to him [mentor] and he'll say, "Rudy, let's think about this." And he gets me thinking in the right direction. I feel like he's known me for years–and that hits me where I live. He's like filling a vacancy I've had in my life for years. And now that my dad is gone, well, he's [mentor] really filling a real void. (Rudy)

I'm always thinking about my father–he's deceased now. He's always in my mind, how I used to be able to confide in him like nobody else. He died after my first head injury. Dr. Murphy [mentor] has sorta filled that hole. I guess I feel grateful for his help. (Sal)

CONTRIBUTING TO OTHERS THROUGH COMMUNITY MEMBER ROLES AND EXTENDED-FAMILY ROLES: "HELPING OTHER PEOPLE IS HELPING MYSELF"

The men also reported that one of the most meaningful experiences that occurred through the intervention was the opportunity to contribute to others through community member and extended-family roles. The men expressed that having the opportunity to help others enabled them to feel a greater sense of competency, usefulness, and personal control.

It means the world to me to be able to help other people. I was always that type a guy, the guy my buddies called on when they got into a jam. I live for helping others. The young kid [extended-family little brother] and I are close, man-to-man and such. I've assisted him in things he wasn't too sure about and things he couldn't physically do. It's positive reinforcement for me. It makes me feel a little bit more like a caring, competent, capable man. Giving helps me feel better about myself. (Rudy)

I feel good when I'm helping the guys [clients] on campus. Then I feel like I have control. I feel like I'm doing what I want to be doing instead of being put somewhere because I'm a client. (Sal)

I always have the fear that I'll take on a challenge and I won't succeed. Getting to help other people is fulfilling because I'm able to do for others and succeed at it. I feel satisfied that I was able to help someone else. (Sal)

I like helping others. I realize that sometimes the best way to help other people is to help myself. But sometimes helping other people is helping myself. It makes me feel good, you know, like I can be useful to someone else and not just ask for help. Like when my sister was going through a lot, getting married, moving. I think I was able to help like an older brother, offer encouragement, tell her I love her, just being supportive. (Jay)

For the two older men in particular, Sal and Rudy, the opportunity to impart their knowledge to others enabled them to feel that their life experience was meaningful beyond their own lives and served to help individuals in the larger society. This sentiment was congruent with Erikson's (1950) life stage of generativity versus stagnation, in which individuals nearing the end of middle age strive to create further meaning in their lives by contributing in significant ways to younger generations.

People always looked up to me. I haven't been in that position in a long time until maybe recently. And now I'm trying to help others as others helped me when I was in that same position. And I'll tell you, when I'm donating my time helping others is when I feel like I'm doing the most good. Because when I was in rehab, I saw how others helped me. It just makes me feel good, you know, to know that I'm able to be of assistance to other people–that I'm giving back some of what was given to me. (Sal)

I love to help [extended-family little brother] getting in and out of the car, up the curb. It's the wind in my sails to help him. I like to relate my experience to him in different ways. You know, I've been on this planet longer than him and I've dealt with the head injury thing for longer than he has. It makes me feel good to help him. Or when I spoke to the students. I can express more of my knowledge and abilities and have them be appreciated by others. It makes me feel like not such a loser. I'm a middle-aged man; I'd like to be able to convey some of the knowledge I've acquired as a 48 year old man whose been living with this head injury for over 20 years now. (Rudy)

FEAR OF STAFF REPRISAL: THE SABOTAGE OF PERSONAL GROWTH

One concern that the men consistently expressed was that although they now perceived their roles to be more congruent with those of an adult man's, the men feared that the direct-care staff members who worked in their community group homes would not support their newly rebuilt independent roles and activities. This concern emerged so frequently in the men's interviews that it became important to consider this finding as an independent thematic category.

I see myself more like an adult man now, but an adult man incarcerated. When I'm with [Rudy's mentor and the therapist who implemented his intervention] that's great–I'm able to do the things and activities like any other adult man. But when I'm here [in the group home] and only [the direct-care staff] are here it's like being in prison. The staff keep a tight rein on all activity. It's stricter than when I was in the Army. And if I mess up or do something wrong–even by accident, accidents happen, I'm only human–the staff take my phone privileges away or they won't walk me to [a local restaurant] to meet friends. Or they say there's no time for it. But I think they just don't wanna be bothered. It's like being grounded when you're an adolescent, you know what I mean? (Rudy)

It's like now I have the reigns in my hands but I don't have no control to go where I want to go. I have more chances to be the man I wanna be but I don't know if the staff people here are gonna let me carry out these things I'm ready to do now independently. Like making phone calls to my friends or going uptown to meet one of the guys. You know like if I wanted to give [client's name] a call and arrange to meet him for dinner at [a local restaurant] there's always a good chance that [a staff member] will can the whole idea. I don't feel like I have any control. The staff take you down avenues that don't go nowhere, they're dead-ends. (Rudy)

I feel like the staff treat me like a child–having to be looked after instead of treated like an adult man. I can't stay over [night] at Ann's house, I have a curfew here. If I want to spend my money on Ann, the staff complain that I'm spending too much money. Or they want me to eat in the group home instead of spending my money to go out to eat. It's miserably ironic. The few things that I have that make me feel like an adult, they're [the staff] trying to see to it that it don't happen. (Sal)

I try to get along with the staff. I know I'm not exactly easy to be around, too. But I feel the staff people are often demeaning and they talk down to me a lot. It's like they give me orders. I know they're probably trying to be helpful but I'm not sure I really feel respected by them most of the time. (Jay)

UNFULFILLED EXPECTATIONS: "THINGS ARE BETTER, BUT . . ."

Additionally, after the intervention Rudy and Sal indicated that they continued to lack specific roles that they believed would have enabled them to feel more like adult men. Rudy, who through his participation in the intervention began to accompany female acquaintances to dinner, expressed disappointment that he had not as yet developed a monogamous sexual relationship with any of the women he had been dating.

Well, it helps to be able to go out with certain lady friends. I mean it makes me feel more like the man I am. But none of em are serious relationships and that hurts, too. It pains me that no one wants to be more than just pals with me. "Hey Rudy, yeah he's a good buddy. He's good to have dinner and a drink with but that's all." I still wish I could have a relationship with a woman and love her and be loved.

Similarly, Sal expressed dissatisfaction with his inability to obtain apartment living.

> I'd feel like a man if I could get back to the apartments and live more independently. I don't feel like an adult in the group home and I resent having to live there. And I resent not having as much privacy with Ann as I think we should be entitled to being two adults.

While the intervention provided greater opportunities for Rudy and Sal to participate in adult male roles, it did not provide sufficient opportunity to transition through specific desired rites of passage into male adulthood. For Rudy, the ability to obtain independent community travel privileges and to develop a monogamous sexual relationship continued to remain elusive. Sal, too, indicated that he could not feel completely satisfied with his post-injury gender role until he had attained apartment living in the community.

Chapter 7

Conclusion:
An Analysis
of the Intervention's Effectiveness

The following is a discussion of the intervention's effectiveness. To determine whether the men's satisfaction with their male gender roles changed as a result of their participation in the intervention, we compared their pre-, concurrent, and post-intervention interviews.

EFFECTIVENESS OF THE INTERVENTION

In their pre-intervention interviews, the four men expressed dissatisfaction with their ability to meet male role expectations and to participate in adult male activities. Specifically, the men reported disappointment that they had neither been able to develop meaningful work nor attain the roles of spouse, father, and friend. For example, in his pre-intervention interview Rudy was able to articulately capture the men's feelings when he expressed, "A part of my life is missing. It's like living somebody else's life. I know it's me. But it doesn't seem like me–I mean the me I thought I'd be as an adult man."

After the intervention, the men's enhanced gender role satisfaction was reflected in the interview theme, "greater satisfaction with post-injury male gender roles." The men described a variety of roles

[Haworth co-indexing entry note]: "Conclusion: An Analysis of the Intervention's Effectiveness." Gutman, Sharon A. Co-published simultaneously in *Occupational Therapy in Mental Health* (The Haworth Press, Inc.) Vol. 15, No. 3/4, 2000, pp. 127-143; and: *Brain Injury and Gender Role Strain: Rebuilding Adult Lifestyles After Injury* (Sharon A. Gutman) The Haworth Press, Inc., 2000, pp. 127-143. Single or multiple copies of this article are available for a fee from The Haworth Document Delivery Service [1-800-342-9678, 9:00 a.m. - 5:00 p.m. (EST). E-mail address: getinfo@haworthpressinc.com].

127

through which they were able to feel more like adult men. Establishing *community member roles*, developing *friendships*, and cultivating *extended-family roles* provided the opportunity for the men to build the relationships through which they could express their male identity in more satisfying ways.

> I feel like an adult again, using the computer to express myself . . . . It feels really good to act in an adult way–to create something that other people seem to respect and value me for. (Jay)

> Being able to walk around the community, meet friends at restaurants, call my friends up [on the phone] makes me feel like an independent adult man. I've wanted to be an independent man. I'm 30. It's about time. (Ed)

> It feels good to get done what I'm supposed to at work. I feel like I'm doing something with my life, like a responsible man. (Ed)

> It's really been important to me to have roles other than just being a client. Being able to go out to dinner with Ann or my role as a client transport at the nursing home. These things have made me feel better about the way I feel about my life now. It feels more like an adult man's [life]. (Sal)

It appears that building *community member roles, friendships,* and *extended-family roles* are essential for men with TBI to feel like adult men. These are roles in which the men believed that they could contribute to others in valuable ways. By making valuable contributions to others, the men expressed that they were more able to feel like adult members of the larger human community.

It was significant that prior to the intervention, the men reported that they had begun to lose a sense of themselves as adult men. Rudy's descriptions below capture the sentiments shared by the four men.

> I don't feel like I'm an adult here, or looked upon as an adult here [in the TBI rehabilitation facility]. I'm treated like an adolescent . . . . I just don't feel like I'm given the chances to act like an adult.

> Being a client with a head injury is a career in itself. And being a client makes your gender neutral. It's like you lose what it's like to be a man.

After the intervention, the men reported that they felt more like the men they used to be prior to injury–a sentiment noted in the interview theme, "feeling like oneself again."

> I'm finally getting back some of me, doing things I though I'd be doing as an adult man. . . . I feel more like the guy I used to be, now, being able to have friends again, or I guess even wanting to be around people again. (Sal)

> I feel more like who I think I really am or could be if given the chance. I'm more in line with the guy I used to imagine I would turn into in my adulthood. (Jay)

> My relationship with Ann makes me feel more normal, cause it reminds me of how I thought of myself as an adult man before my accident. (Sal)

The men may have been able to experience greater gender role satisfaction after the intervention because they were able to establish a greater congruency between their image of themselves as men and their actual opportunities to enact desired male roles.

It was noteworthy also, that several of the men reported that through their participation in the intervention they were able to demonstrate to family members that they had achieved certain expected male gender roles–a significant finding as the men initially reported feeling dissatisfied with their ability to meet parental expectations for an adult male lifestyle. These pre-intervention sentiments were articulately expressed by Rudy and Jay.

> I know my dad would have wanted me to lead a different life . . . . I know I'm a disappointment to him. I feel real bad about that. I really want my dad to see me a little more stable and competent–more like the man I know I can be–before he passes away. (Rudy)

> Sometimes it's hard for me to deal with the feeling that I haven't measured up. . . . I don't want my mom and stepdad to feel burdened with my care the rest of their lives. As an adult I'd like to be self-supporting. (Jay)

The above comments contrast sharply with the men's post-intervention statements regarding their ability to participate in male gender roles that were congruent with perceived parental expectations.

> Now I can show my parents that I'm an adult man. I have friends and a girlfriend. I work. I can take my own money and go out to eat with friends. (Ed)

> I felt my dad got a chance to glimpse the real me before his death–I mean, to see me more like the man I feel myself to be. . . . I think he got a chance to say, "Yeah, that's my son Rudy, the man I knew he could be." (Rudy)

> I want my family to see the productive side of me, that I can be more independent and not burden my parents as much. I think my mom was surprised but also proud to see me be writing again. (Jay)

The ability to meet perceived parental expectations appeared to be a strong motivating factor in the men's rehabilitation. The men expressed guilt for having forced their parents to become caregivers, and for failing to live up to parental expectations. Such feelings of guilt and failure were likely deeply seated in each man's psyche and difficult to resolve. The opportunity to resolve such parental conflicts appears to be another critical factor underlying the alleviation of gender role strain. When an individual is unable to resolve conflicts with his actual parents (perhaps because of death or geographical separation), extended-family and/or mentors can sometimes assume the parental relationship and help the individual to resolve long-existing conflicts. *Confirmation from a parent that one has indeed rebuilt an adult male lifestyle after TBI is often an important aspect involved in the alleviation of gender role strain, albeit a difficult one to attain.*

The incongruence between one's own personal expectations for an adult male lifestyle and one's current life as a client in a TBI facility, may be even more difficult to resolve. Both Sal and Jay were able to exemplify the men's regret that they had not met personal expectations for an adult male lifestyle after injury.

> I haven't met the expectations I had for myself. I might have met them for a short time previously–before my accident–but no more. (Sal)

> I'm not the adult I could have been if things were different. (Jay)

Based on the men's post-intervention self-reports, it appears that the ability to rebuild and meet long-term goals that had remained elusive after injury, can significantly enhance an individual's gender role satisfaction. This was reflected in the post-intervention theme, "attaining personal goals," in which the men expressed that their ability to achieve long-held adult life goals reduced the discrepancy between their pre- and post-injury self-concept as an adult man.

> It seemed like I would never write again. . . . I'm fulfilling my expectations pretty much now. I'm feeding myself with fulfillment with goals I had for myself. (Jay)

> I'm more comfortable now with talking to women. I'm shy; it used to be hard for me to talk to women. . . . Now I can hold a conversation with a woman. . . . I always wanted to be able to talk more easy with women like other guys. (Ed)

> Well, I wanted to date again [after his TBI] but I never seemed to have luck with women. . . . I guess I'm lucky to have met Ann. I didn't think it [developing a dating relationship] would happen, but I'm glad it did. (Sal)

> Just hanging out with the guys. . . . You don't know how good that is for me–to have that [role] back in my life, being a man's man. I wanted that for a long time. (Rudy)

Additionally, the men indicated that the intervention provided the opportunity to rebuild *three primary life values* into their post-injury adult lives–*volitional control, competency,* and *normalcy.*

Volitional Control: "A Freshman in College Forever"

Initially, the men expressed that being a client in a community group home had diminished their ability to exercise choice.

> I don't feel particularly autonomous here in a community group home. It's kind of like being a freshman in college forever. You don't choose where to live or who to live with. You're assigned your classes–but here [rehabilitation facility] it's your therapies. You have specific meal times and you can't choose what to eat.

> When I used to live by myself I could do the things that, you know, made you feel like an autonomous adult. Like if I wanted to grab a sandwich and a beer and put my feet up and watch a ball game. You can't do that here.

After the intervention, the men reported having greater opportunities to act upon their volition and to exercise choice–a characteristic of an adult lifestyle that was highly valued by the participants and served to enhance their post-injury gender role satisfaction.

> You never get to make a decision about how to spend your time–what activities to do [as a client]. But now that's changed to some degree. I can't even express to you what a change in life-style this is, having some ability to see friends or take a lady out to dinner. It's normal, like any other person in society. (Rudy)

> I feel good when I'm helping the guys [clients] on campus [in Sal's role as an extended-family big brother]. Then I feel like I have control. I feel like I'm doing what I want to be doing instead of being put somewhere because I'm a client. (Sal)

> I feel more in control of my life. I'm doing the things adults do. I am an adult. I have a social life like an adult man now. Before [the intervention period] I didn't. I didn't have any friends. I didn't talk to people much. (Ed)

> I still don't feel totally autonomous living here [in the community group home] but I can see where I can exercise adult control over my own pursuits and things I'd like to do. It makes me feel more in control, like a responsible adult. (Jay)

Competency as a "Caring and Capable Man"

The ability to feel greater competency in one's role as an adult man was a second strongly held value that the men were able to rebuild after intervention. Competency was both highly regarded by the men and contributed to feelings of greater life purpose and meaning.

> It means the world to me to be able to help other people [through community member roles]. . . . It's positive reinforcement for

me. It makes me feel a little bit more like a caring, competent, and capable man. (Rudy)

Having more friends, writing again–this brings out a feeling of competence. I want my family to see the productive side of me, that I can be more independent and not burden my parents as much. (Jay)

People always looked up to me. I haven't been in that position in a long time until maybe recently. And now I'm trying to help others as others helped me when I was in that same position. . . . Getting to help other people is fulfilling because I'm able to do for others and succeed at it. (Sal)

I love to help [extended-family little brother] getting in and out of the car, up the curb. . . . Or when I spoke to the students. I can express more of my knowledge and abilities and have them be appreciated by others. It makes me feel like not such a loser. I'm a middle-aged man; I'd like to be able to convey some of the knowledge I've acquired as a 48 year old man who's been living with this head injury for over 20 years now. (Rudy)

Normalcy: "Like a Member of Society"

A third highly valued lifestyle change that the men were able to effect was their ability to rebuild a sense of normalcy into their everyday lives. The men expressed that through the rebuilding of desired male gender roles and activities they were able to feel more like any other person in the larger society–a value noted in the post-intervention theme, "feeling more like a member of society."

It's made such a difference, being able to go up town [in the community], up to the shopping center, have dinner with friends . . . . I'm just about at a point where I feel like I'm stepping into being a societal member again. (Rudy)

It's nice to be out in public, doing things like a normal citizen. Doing things it takes to live like a normal person–normal things which seem small, but which are very big and basic parts of life in our society. Like maybe meeting friends for a meal or seeing a movie together. (Jay)

> I feel for the first time that I'm accepted here. I don't feel like everyone hates me anymore. That means so much to me because I always wanted to have friends like normal people. (Jay)

Volitional control, competency, and normalcy are three aspects that appear necessary for men with TBI to feel some degree of personal life satisfaction. They are factors that also appear to be necessary for one to feel a sense of adulthood. Volitional control, competency, and normalcy had remained absent from the men's lives since injury. The ability to regain (a) volitional control over everyday decisions, (b) competency in meaningful life skills, and (c) normalcy in one's everyday routine enabled each man to experience his identity as an adult man.

MEANINGFUL ROLES IN VALUED RELATIONSHIPS

It is interesting to note that of the six roles addressed in the intervention (familial, extended-family, friend, dating/courtship, mentor-protégé, and community member), the men reported that five of the roles held the most personal meaning: *dating/courtship, mentor-protégé, community member, friend, and extended-family roles.* Familial roles were not identified by the men as having the same importance as the five other roles.

The opportunity to develop a relationship with a male mentor having knowledge of the head injury experience and who could serve as a guide was a novel experience for each of the four men. In fact, male mentors were often conspicuously absent from several of the men's pre-injury lives.

> My father didn't have much to do with me. He'd spend a lot of time with my brothers but not me. I never knew why. I thought there musta been something wrong with me. . . . My brothers and I weren't close. They did their own things. They played softball with my dad but not me. (Ed)

> It's been so many years of distance where we haven't been father and son. I don't feel that I know him [stepfather] at all. . . . My real father excommunicated me after my accident. I feel bad about that. (Jay)

The men expressed that through their participation in the intervention they were able to forge relationships with male mentors who provided guidance, acceptance, and a feeling of being understood–all experiences which the men considered to be highly meaningful. The opportunity to feel accepted and understood by a male mentor was reported to be a unique post-injury experience for the men who, in their pre-intervention interviews, expressed that they felt ostracized and alienated from prominent men in their lives after TBI.

> I never really had a real father or a brother, you know, someone I could sort of turn to for male advice. It's nice to have someone to fill that need. (Jay)

> I feel like he's [mentor] known me for years–and that hits me where I live. He's filling a vacancy I've had in my life for years. And now that my dad is gone, well he's [mentor] really filling a real void. (Rudy)

> I finally found the man I've been looking for to model myself after his image and intelligence for the last 20 years. [Mentor's name] understands me to a tee. He knows exactly what I'm trying to say when I'm trying to describe what it's like for me in some such situation because of this head injury. . . . I feel completely accepted by him. He doesn't look at me like I'm from another planet–like so many other people do. (Rudy)

> I consider [mentor's name] to be one of my closest friends here [at the facility]. I can talk to him like a friend, like the friends I used to have in high school. (Ed)

> [Mentor's name] is like a friend to me. He treats me with respect like I'm a grown man and he doesn't talk down to me like the other staff people. I don't feel like I'm just a client with him. He respects my experience and that I had a life before this head injury. And I respect him for that because with him I feel like a whole man, not some freak. (Sal)

Similarly, the men reported that the opportunity to build friendships with peers who could provide a sense of shared experience and affinity was strongly appreciated. The ability to confide in a peer who demonstrated understanding and acceptance helped the men to feel a greater sense of personal comfort with their post-injury roles as adult men.

[Male client] and I share a similar life experience and mental knowledge of what it's like to be a 50 year old man with a head injury. . . . It feels great to talk to someone who understands what I'm talking about. . . . I don't feel so much like the odd ball from mars with [client's name].

Ann is a good friend that I'm able to be myself with. We're both disabled, we have this in common. We're two disabled people that society looks upon and points a finger at. So in that respect she knows what it's like to be head injured. I enjoy her company and I feel like she knows me well and accepts me for who I am. (Sal)

I've really gotten significantly tight and close with [male client]. And it's always nice to have someone going through the same thing as whatever you're going through. . . . Having someone I can feel like-minded with. . . . It's a gift from God to be able to find someone who knows what I'm going through. (Rudy)

Another significant role that was lacking from the men's post-injury lives was a dating/courtship role. The men reported in their pre-intervention interviews that their primary opportunity to interact with women came from relationships with female direct-care staff members.

The female staff here at [name of facility] act like my mother. I don't feel like an adult man. I feel talked down to. (Sal)

Finding women here [inside of the residential TBI facility] is like trying to find water in a desert. I used to date a lot. Now I feel like a penned up stag. What am I supposed to say to some lady I may meet outside of [facility's name]? Come over to my group home?

After the intervention, the men reported that having the opportunity to socialize with female companions and to develop dating relationships, significantly contributed to their enhanced feelings of gender role satisfaction–perhaps more than any other role.

It means the world to me to be able to have dinner with a lady friend. Or to talk on the phone with a woman. Before my accident I had a really active social life, you know what I'm saying? It was like having my left arm cut off, being here, being restricted from women. Or really like having some other body appendage cut off, you know what I'm saying? It's made a big difference being able to socialize and such with ladies. That's the kinda man I am. I need this [socializing with women] to feel like myself, like the man I am. (Rudy)

I've enjoyed having dinner with [several female clients]. It's fun, like I guess how dating is sort of. I wouldn't know–I didn't really date a lot before my injury. But now I think I can talk more easily now–I mean with women. I like that about myself; it's cool. (Jay)

I'm not seeing Arlene but we write every week. I like her and I know she likes me too. We're more than just friends. I feel like I have a girlfriend now. I'm happy. I wanted a girlfriend for a long time. (Ed)

I'm glad we can have this part of our relationship together [sexual experiences]. . . . It makes me feel more normal, like the person I used to be. And I want Ann to get a chance to see the real me, not just the head injured part of me. (Sal)

Each of the men also reported that having the opportunity to contribute to others through community member and extended-family roles substantially enhanced their satisfaction with post-injury gender roles.

I definitely feel like I have more responsibilities now than at any other time since my accident. And yeah, that's a pretty good feeling. But I would imagine it would make anybody feel good to have a life where they were doing things, meaningful things; not just sitting around. At least I'd rather be active and have adult responsibilities. . . . My volunteer job in [the nursing home] and here [in the crafts group], I guess let's me be responsible for others. And helping others really is the only time when I feel completely separate from being a client, like I'm not a client anymore; it's like I'm a man like any other man. (Sal)

When I'm donating my time helping others is when I feel like I'm doing the most good. Because when I was in rehab I saw how others helped me. It just makes me feel good, you know, to know that I'm able to be of assistance to other people [as an extended-family big-brother and community member]–that I'm giving back some of what was given to me. (Sal)

Speaking to the students gave me a chance to impart the knowledge I've acquired as a forty-some year old man with head injury to others. It made me feel like, yeah, I do have something of importance to say that will help other people. I felt like the wise man I know myself to be deep inside. It made me feel important, like people valued what I could say about living with a head injury for twenty-some years. (Rudy)

Mentor, friend, extended-family member, dating/courtship, and community member roles appeared to hold considerable meaning for the men, perhaps because these were roles through which the men reported receiving personal acceptance as adult men. Conversely, already established familial roles were less frequently considered as important to the men's enhanced post-injury gender role satisfaction–perhaps because such roles were often conflicted and laden with prior disappointments. Nevertheless, for Jay and Rudy, the opportunity to contribute to family members as a brother and an uncle was meaningful and enabled them to feel more satisfied in desired familial roles.

It makes me feel good, you know, like I can be useful to someone else and not just ask for help. Like when my sister was going through a lot, you know, getting married, moving. I think I was able to help like an older brother, offer encouragement, tell her I love her, just being supportive. (Jay)

I think [the role of] being a brother is a lot more satisfying to me now, maybe more than it ever was, or at least since I can remember. I feel accepted as a brother now. I feel like, yeah, I *am* [his emphasis] a brother. That feels really good. (Jay)

Now I'm actually giving something back to my family through the younger generation of [family's surname]. I always saw myself as the generous Italian-American uncle who could give my nieces and nephews my knowledge or you know slip them a five [dollar bill] now and then. And now I'm making them toys and such. . . . It makes me feel a real part of the family in a good way. You know, not just asking for help most of the time. I want to be able to give something back. (Rudy)

In contrast, Sal's ability to participate in desired male gender roles helped him to feel liberated from his conflicted relationship with his mother.

My socialization is much more personally satisfying now since I've been seeing Ann and becoming friends with [several male clients]. Mother's negative actions and words don't seem to bother me as much; well, I'm not really having as much contact with her as I used to. . . . I guess I don't feel that I need her so much; I mean I don't feel as much by myself as I did. . . . I've learned there are people in this world who can be trusted, I think. I don't have to keep knocking my head against a wall trying to have a relationship with Mother if it isn't gonna be there.

MEANINGFUL ACTIVITIES

The men were also able to identify the activities that most effectively supported the acquisition of new post-injury male gender roles. In their pre-intervention interviews, the men indicated that most of their post-injury activities were ones that supported their role as a client living in a community group home. Such activities included completing community group home chores, maintaining the personal room in the group home, and attending to health maintenance needs secondary to TBI. Activities that supported the role of a client, however, did not support the role of an adult man. Other activities in which the men participated that were unrelated to the client role only served to facilitate isolation (e.g., watching television or listening to music alone in one's room). These activities neither preserved participation in pre-injury male gender roles nor supported the acquisition of new post-injury roles.

As a result of their participation in the intervention, the men indicated that they gained the opportunity to engage in activities that supported their roles as adult men. *Activities that enabled the men to create adult male lifestyles characterized by volitional control, competency, and normalcy were most valued.* For example, the ability to participate in activities that facilitated a sense of *volitional control* was reported to hold considerable meaning for the men.

> When I'm painting or making toys for my nephews and nieces–sitting on the back deck with my Yanni tapes plugged in–I feel I'm in my own world. A world where I'm in control and nobody makes the decisions but me. (Rudy)

> Writing takes me any place I wanna go, you know what I mean? I mean not literally but symbolically. I can create the atmosphere when I write. I can create a better place to be if I'm not happy being in my present place. Nobody else can interfere or tell me what to do when I write. It's all totally up to me only. (Jay)

> I felt proud. Everybody saw me running the [Goldfish Throw] booth at Visitor's Day. I was in charge for once. People came to me for help. I knew I could do it. (Ed)

Activities that enabled the men to feel more *competent* in their roles as adult men were also highly regarded.

> Writing has helped me to get to know myself better. It's changed the way I see myself. I see myself now as intelligent, curious, interested, and motivated to improve myself and make the most of my assets. I have greater self-confidence now. (Jay)

> I feel like an adult again, using the computer to express myself. I didn't think I'd write again after my accident. It feels really good to act in an adult way–to create something that other people seem to respect and value me for. (Jay)

> I can't tell you how happy I am to get down on my hands and knees in the dirt and tend a living plant that I know is only gonna survive if I take care of it. . . . It's a wonderful thing to be able to grow something with your own sweat and blood that is appreciated by others. When me and [staff member's name] cook my tomatoes into a sauce and we eat it with spaghetti or have them in a salad I feel like the world is smiling. (Rudy)

> I feel like I'm doing something with my mind and my hands [in the ceramics class] instead of just sitting around [name of facility]. I'm doing something to increase my mental stimulation. . . . It feels good to be amongst other people who are just as inter-

ested in improving their knowledge and experience and lot in life like I am. (Rudy)

Similarly, the men also valued activities that facilitated a greater sense of *normalcy* in their everyday lives.

I think it's normal to be able to call your friends or see a movie or go out to dinner with your girlfriend. But when you're a client you don't have those activities to do–you have client activities. "Clean you room Rudy. Put your dishes in the sink, Rudy. Take your meds, Rudy." It's insane. It's made a real difference, being able to do normal things. Going up town [in the community] to have dinner with friends. Asking a lady out for a nice Friday night dinner. I'm walking the line of being closer to being in society. It's like I'm starting to step over that line into society again. (Rudy)

Everything's regulated here [at the rehabilitation facility]. Everything here revolves around being a client. It's nice to be able to do something that has nothing to do with being a client. Writing, going to movies with a friend, going on a date. It feels normal. It's more like living like any normal person lives. (Jay)

It is an important observation that the men primarily identified gender-neutral activities as important to their adult male gender role satisfaction. It appeared more important for the activities to facilitate feelings of control, competency, and normalcy, than to possess a traditional masculine identification.

STAFF CONFLICT WITH THE MEN'S NEWLY REBUILT ROLES AND ACTIVITIES

One disconcerting finding of the study related to the men's fear that the direct-care staff members would not support the men's newly rebuilt roles and activities. In their post-intervention interviews several of the men indicated that staff members had been unable or unwilling to provide the assistance necessary for a man to enact a desired role (e.g., accompaniment into the community, or assistance to make phone calls). Several of the men stated that newly gained activities supporting male gender roles had been revoked on occasion in response to behavior considered to be inappropriate (for example, Rudy reported that his phone privileges were often retracted). As a result, the men reported feeling uncertain that their greater sense of volitional control would continue once the intervention period ended.

The intervention was intended to provide the men with the assistance needed to rebuild and enact adult male gender roles. While we provided such assistance during the period of intervention, it was hoped that the direct-care staff members would assume that responsibility once the intervention formally ended. However, rather than considering the intervention to be a therapeutic part of the men's rehabilitation, it appeared instead that the direct-care staff members perceived the intervention to be a recreational privilege–one that could be revoked if the men's behavior conflicted with norms in the community group home.

It became apparent that the intervention actually conflicted with the larger culture of the facility's community group home program. In the culture of the group home it appeared that a hierarchy existed between the staff members and the clients, similar to the hierarchy between officers and enlisted men in the Army. Direct-care staff members were often the employees who were the least educated and the least paid. They often misunderstand the philosophy underlying rehabilitation–that rehabilitation is the process by which individuals with disabilities are assisted to regain optimal independence in all daily living activities. Instead, direct-care staff members often assumed a parental-like attitude of over-protection. Such attitudes were reflected in statements such as, "What I say goes," "I'm in charge, not you," and "This is for your own good." Unspoken norms appeared to characterize staff-client interactions. For example, as noted previously, most patterns of communication existed within one-to-one interactions between a client and staff member. Client-to-client interactions were often interrupted and stopped by staff members–who may have adopted this strategy to maintain a measure of control by preventing client-client disruptions before they occurred. Unfortunately, this pattern of communication neither encouraged the clients to gain the skills necessary to build peer relationships nor to independently resolve conflicts. It became increasingly apparent that the client behaviors that were encouraged by the staff members in the group home setting did not enable the men to feel like adult men. In fact, some of the staff-to-client interactions actually appeared to inhibit client independence and competence. It sometimes seemed as though the staff members enjoyed exercising power over the clients, as it was not uncommon for staff members to revoke client privileges for what seemed to be only minimal transgressions.

While the intervention appeared to effectively help the men to enhance their own adult male gender performance skills, the larger culture of the group home environment did not appear to support the men's greater independence and competence. It became necessary to provide greater education to the direct-care staff to help them learn how to empower clients and facilitate their identity as adult men.

In summary, it appears that helping men with TBI to rebuild adult lifestyles is best facilitated by the following factors:

- Provide the opportunity for the individual to rebuild *community member, mentor-protégé, friend, extended-family,* and *dating/ courtship roles*. These are roles through which others can demonstrate their acceptance of the individual as an adult man.
- When possible, help the individual to rebuild already established *familial roles*. Caution in rebuilding familial roles is warranted, as familial roles may be laden with conflict and prior disappointment.
- Provide the opportunity for the individual to rebuild *roles through which he can contribute to others in valued ways*. Contributing to the larger community facilitates feelings of being appreciated and feelings of usefulness. Community member roles, friendships, and extended-family roles often allow the individual to contribute to others in valuable ways that promote feelings of belonging and group membership.
- While familial roles may be difficult to rebuild–when it is possible–the opportunity to *demonstrate to parents that the individual has assumed adult male roles* appears to facilitate gender role satisfaction.
- Provide the opportunity for the individual to *meet personal gender role expectations for an adult male lifestyle*. When individuals are able to meet personal goals–for which they gave up hope post-injury–gender role satisfaction is greatly facilitated.
- Provide the opportunity for the individual to rebuild a sense of *volitional control, competency, and normalcy* back into his adult life through desired male gender roles and activities. These are characteristics of an adult lifestyle.
- Provide education for *direct-care staff and all caregivers* to learn how to facilitate the man's independence and sense of personal life control.

Epilogue:
My Final Thoughts

As a therapist I felt a multitude of emotions during and after the four months in which I worked with Rudy, Sal, Ed, and Jay. It was both rewarding and hopeful to see these men rebuild roles and relationships through which they derived greater life satisfaction as adult men. I felt elated when Ed visited his girlfriend in another state and experienced his first "real date" shortly after the intervention ended. It was gratifying to see Jay engaged in the writing of a book about his injury experience–a creative endeavor that allowed the expression of his high level intelligence, which was otherwise disguised in a body that was listless and slow. I cheered when I heard that Sal and Ann had celebrated one-half a year together, three months after the intervention came to a completion. And I felt triumphant when Rudy's paintings and jewelry were displayed in the main lobby of his rehabilitation facility the following fall. His family came to that event–an exhibition of his artwork and jewelry that had come to define a new adult identity for him.

I also experienced sadness and distress when Jay's house staff denied him access to his computer as a punishment for refusing to shower one night. Or when Rudy's phone privileges were retracted by a staff member for arguing with another male client who shared his residence. I felt defeated when I would go to the group homes to work with one of the men and the staff would inform me that I "was going to ruin the men's morale by giving them false hope. They're starting to believe that they can do anything they want, just like the rest of us [non-clients]. Don't they know they have serious problems?" At another group home I was

[Haworth co-indexing entry note]: "Epilogue: My Final Thoughts." Gutman, Sharon A. Co-published simultaneously in *Occupational Therapy in Mental Health* (The Haworth Press, Inc.) Vol. 15, No. 3/4, 2000, pp. 145-147; and: *Brain Injury and Gender Role Strain: Rebuilding Adult Lifestyles After Injury* (Sharon A. Gutman) The Haworth Press, Inc., 2000, pp. 145-147. Single or multiple copies of this article are available for a fee from The Haworth Document Delivery Service [1-800-342-9678, 9:00 a.m. - 5:00 p.m. (EST). E-mail address: getinfo@haworthpressinc.com].

told that I "shouldn't encourage the clients to go to each other's houses for visits cause it burdens the staff to have to look after another one of 'em." Another staff member helpfully advised me that Rudy was "getting one over on [me] by making all these phone calls. Who does he need to call? He doesn't know anyone."

While some of the staff members were genuine in their concern for the men and created a loving and compassionate environment in which the men could thrive, the attitudes of several other staff members made me feel as though I was an unwanted intruder who had come to destroy the peace and order of their group home culture. All the while I smiled and tried to explain that these men could be more independent, more socially adept, more like us even. I knew that by challenging certain staff members I risked alienating them–and the reality was that I needed their support for the intervention methods to be effective. I needed the staff to help the men by continuing to use the therapeutic strategies that I would no longer be able to implement once the four months were finished and I left the facility to resume former work.

There can be an unpleasant phenomenon that occurs simply by placing humans in a position of power over other humans. We sometimes take our roles of authority too seriously and exaggerate the need for control in an effort to maintain order. The staff may have feared that earlier behaviors that the clients exhibited–which were destructive– may return if the men were afforded greater independence. Perhaps the staff feared that their own jobs would become jeopardized if the men required less staff supervision. Some may even have enjoyed the authority afforded by their work, finding that it was one area of their lives in which they could exert control.

As a therapist, I changed as a result of my experience with these four men. I learned that we are no more competent than our environment allows us to be. As health care professionals, occupational therapists aim to change the way in which the individual interacts with his or her environment in order to promote competence. People who work in health care are not gatekeepers to the path of health. We are not shepherds herding passive sheep to greener pastures. Our role is more similar to the gardener who prunes dead branches, braces a weak tree trunk in the winter, and waters the tree's roots during a dry spell. Like the gardener, our goal is to make a weak tree stronger so that eventually the tree will continue growing in its natural environment without our further intervention. If we are lucky, the tree will thrive in its surroundings and contribute valuable resources to an ecosystem in which all beings benefit.

I tried to encourage several of the staff members to understand that by helping these men to lead more independent, satisfying adult lives, the staff would benefit also. I reasoned that even if several members of the staff were unable to consider that all humans gain by encouraging the perceived weaker among us to become whole–to live actualized, full lives–at least the staff could understand that as employed workers they would have less work if the men were empowered to create adult lives, rich with activities that fostered competency, personal control, and normalcy. As individuals who work in health care, and as family members and guardians of individuals with disabilities, this is all we can hope for: that we can empower those who enlist our assistance to lead lives of competency, personal control, and normalcy.

Rudy, Sal, Ed, and Jay began to rebuild adult lives in which they felt a greater sense of competency, personal control, and normalcy. But their journey is only at an initial threshold and far from complete. It is my hope that these men will continue to benefit from the assistance of other gardeners who will use the treatment practices described in this book to empower the men to further their growth as adult individuals. It is also my hope–and the hope of Rudy, Sal, Ed, and Jay–that other gardeners will learn from the men's experience and will use the intervention methods to assist more individuals with brain injury to create lives full with activities, roles, and relationships that promote meaningful and satisfying adult lives.

References

Barrett, C. J. (1978). Effectiveness of widow's groups in facilitating change. *Journal of Consulting and Clinical Psychology, 46*, 20-31.

Bem, S. L. (1993). *The lenses of gender.* New Haven, CT: Yale University Press.

Bowen, A., Neumann, V., Conner, M., Tennant, A., & Chamberlain, M. A. (1998). Mood disorders following traumatic brain injury: Identifying the extent of the problem and the people at risk. *Brain Injury, 12*(3), 177-190.

Brain Injury Association. (1997). *Fact Sheet.* Washington, DC: Author.

Brown, M., & Vandergoot, D. (1998). Quality of life for individuals with traumatic brain injury: Comparison with others living in the community. *Journal of Head Trauma Rehabilitation, 13*(4), 1-23.

Brzuzy, S., & Speziale, B. A. (1997). Persons with traumatic brain injuries and their families: Living arrangements and well-being post-injury. *Social Work in Health Care, 26*(1), 77-88.

Burleigh, S. A., Farber, R. S., & Gillard, M. (1998). Community integration and life satisfaction after traumatic brain injury: Long-term findings. *American Journal of Occupational Therapy, 52*(1), 45-52.

Corrigan, J. D., Smith-Knapp, K., & Granger, C. V. (1998). Outcomes in the first 5 years after traumatic brain injury. *Archives of Physical Medicine and Rehabilitation, 79*(3), 298-305.

Davies, D. (1994). Raising the issues. In J. Holm (Ed.), *Rites of passage* (pp. 41-65). New York: St. Martin's Press.

Diasio-Serrett, K., Schallert, R., & Shively, C. S. (1994, July). *Using rites of passage and ritual in therapeutic practice.* Workshop presented at the Canadian-American Occupational Therapy Conference, Boston.

Erikson, E. (1950). *Childhood and society.* New York: W. W. Norton.

Fleming, J., & Strong, J. (1999). A longitudinal study of self-awareness: Functional deficits underestimated by persons with brain injury. *Occupational Therapy Journal of Research, 19*(1), 3-17.

Francel, P. C., & Snell, B. E. (1999). Age and outcome of brain injury. *Brain Injury Source, 3*(1), 8-11.

Geschwind, N., & Galaburda, A. M. (1987). *Cerebral lateralization: Biological mechanisms, associations, and pathology.* Cambridge, MA: MIT Press.

Gomez-Hernandez, R., Max, J. E., Kosier, T., Paradiso, S., & Robinson, R. G. (1997). Social impairment and depresssion after traumatic brain injury. *Archives of Physical Medicine and Rehabilitation, 78*(12), 1321-1326.

Grimes, R. L. (1995). *Marrying and burying: Rites of passage in a man's life.* Boulder, CO: Westview Press.

Gutman, S. A. (1997). Enhancing gender role satisfaction in adult males with traumatic brain injury: A set of guidelines for occupational therapy practice. *Occupational Therapy in Mental Health, 13*(4), 25-43.

Gutman, S. A. (1999). Alleviating gender role strain in adult men with traumatic brain injury: An evaluation of a set of guidelines for occupational therapy. *American Journal of Occupational Therapy, 53*(1), 101-110.

Gutman, S. A., & Napier-Klemic, J. (1996). The impact of head injury on gender identity and gender role. *American Journal of Occupational Therapy, 50,* 535-544.

Jordan, J. V., Kaplan, A. G., Miller, J. B., Stiver, I. P., & Surrey, J. L. (1991). *Women's growth in connection: Writings from the Stone Center.* New York: Guilford Press.

Kaschak, E. (1992). *Engendered lives: A new psychology of women's experience.* New York: Basic Books.

Levinson, D. (1978). *The seasons of a man's life.* New York: Alfred A. Knopf.

Lindsey, L. L. (1994). *Gender roles: A sociological perspective.* Englewood Cliffs, NJ: Prentice-Hall.

Mazaux, J. M., Masson, F., Levin, H. S., Alaoui, P., Maurette, P., & Barat, M. (1997). Long-term neuropsychological outcome and loss of social autonomy after traumatic brain injury. *Archives of Physical Medicine and Rehabilitation, 78*(12), 1316-1320.

Merritt, L. (1999). Relationship issues in traumatic brain injury. *Brain Injury Source, 3*(1), 12-18.

Miller, L. (1990). *Inner natures: Brain, self, and personality.* New York: St. Martin's Press.

Miller, L. (1993). *Psychotherapy of the brain-injured patient: Reclaiming the shattered self.* New York: W. W. Norton.

Money, J. (1994). The concept of gender identity disorder in childhood and adolescence after 39 years. *Journal of Sex and Marital Therapy, 20*(3), 163-177.

Moore, A. D., Stambrook, M., & Gill, D. G. (1994). Coping patterns associated with long-term outcome from traumatic brain injury among female survivors. *Neurorehabilitation, 4*(2), 122-129.

Rosenthal, M., Christensen, B. K., & Ross, T. P. (1998). Depression following traumatic brain injury. *Archives of Physical Medicine and Rehabilitation, 79*(1), 90-103.

Schmidt, M. F., Garvin, L. J., Heinemann, A. W., & Kelley, J. P. (1995). Gender- and age-related role changes following brain injury. *Journal of Head Trauma Rehabilitation, 10,* 14-27.

Trombly, C. A., Radomski, M. V., & Davis, E. S. (1998). Achievement of self-identified goals by adults with traumatic brain injury. *American Journal of Occupational Therapy, 52*(10), 810-818.

Yalom, I. D. (1970). *The theory and practice of group psychotherapy.* New York: Basic Books.

Index

Page numbers followed by *t* indicate tables; those followed by *fig* indicate figures.

Printed in the United States
by Baker & Taylor Publisher Services